To those who need it most,
HOSPICE MEANS HOPE

To those who need it most,
HOSPICE MEANS HOPE

Kenneth B. Wentzel

Charles River Books

Boston

1981

Library of Congress Cataloging in Publication Data

Wentzel, Kenneth B
  To those who need it most, hospice means hope.

  1. Terminal care. 2. Terminal care facilities.
I. Title.
R726.8.W46   362.1'96029   80-21664
ISBN 0-89182-020-5
ISBN 0-89182-030-2 (pbk)

Published by Charles River Books, Inc.
One Thompson Square, Boston, Massachusetts 02129
Copyright 1981 by Charles River Books, Inc.

Ted Rosenthal's poem reprinted from *How Could I Not Be Among You?* by Ted Rosenthal by permission of the publisher, George Braziller, Inc. Copyright 1973 by Ted Rosenthal.

No part of this book may be reproduced in any form by any means, electronic or mechanical, including photocopying and recording, or by any information or storage or retrieval system, without written permission from the publisher, except for brief passages quoted by a reviewer.

ISBN 0 89182 020 5   ISBN 0 89182 030 2 (pbk)
Library of Congress Card Number 80-21664
Printed in the United States of America

To
Robert J. Barden

Preface

A new way of caring for the terminally ill and their families is finding expression in the American health care industry. It is called HOSPICE.

Hospice means that the largely ignored dying cancer patient and his family are being rediscovered and cared for.

To caregivers, hospice means a new kind of team discipline and approach and a broader application of "health care."

To the users of its services, present and future, hospice means that families will no longer need to sit by helplessly and watch a loved one slowly and painfully die of cancer.

To the users of its services, hospice means that when all treatment of the disease ends, caring for the patient and the family increases.

To those people hospice means that no cancer patient need endure the agonies of chronic pain.

And finally, hospice means that concern for the family continues into their time of bereavement.

Some of the ingredients in hospice, such as the control of chronic pain, are new. Other elements—spiritual, psychological, social, and emotional support—are as old as human caring itself. What is radically new to our 20th century culture is the sensitive application of skill and compassion to the total needs of the whole person. Further, this same skill and compassion continues long after aggressive treatment of the disease has ended.

Hospice Means Hope is primarily for those people who may someday be the recipients of hospital care. The book is designed to introduce hospice to the general population in lay terminology, and to explain how hospice works and what can be expected of its caregivers.

Hospice is an idea whose time has arrived. It is not another medical fad; it is here to stay. Its premise and its promise and its performance are so accurately on target in critical health care areas of need that the movement is spreading rapidly.

The National Hospice Organization was formed in October of 1978, in Washington, D.C. Conference planners had optimistically expected four hundred persons to attend. However, over one thousand interested people showed up. They represented over two hundred hospice groups in the United States and Canada, many of them in the formative stages. People who had dreamed the dream of hospice took heart. And Congress took notice. One of the featured speakers, Senator Edward Kennedy of Massachusetts, echoed what all the delegates and their myriad colleagues back home knew and believed. "Hospice is a lot of things," he said, "But most of all, it is a return to humane health care."

CONTENTS

Preface	vii
Introduction	xi
Hospice: A Definition	1
Hospice: Health Care Bridge	11
Control of Chronic Pain	19
Realism About Death	27
"Family" as the Primary Unit of Caring	43
Staff Support	57
Hospice Volunteers	81
Some Final Thoughts About Hospice in America	103

Introduction

For twenty-five years I had been a parish minister, serving three churches in Indiana, Maryland, and Rhode Island. The people of Kingston, Rhode Island Congregational Church had generously included a sabbatical leave in their offer when they invited me to be their minister in 1966.

When the time for sabbatical planning arrived, I had decided to pursue study and service opportunities in caring for the terminally ill. My goals were modest, far more modest than I could ever have thought. I wanted to learn some skills and to gain some knowledge that would help me be a better parish minister. The actual outcome thrust me far beyond those original modest goals. I never dreamed I would become actively involved in the formation of local hospice programs and educational workshops of the National Hospice Organization, let alone write a book on hospice.

I decided to contact St. Christopher's Hospice, London, a pioneer institution in the care of the terminally ill. At first, the lovely lilt of that name conjured up a peaceful medieval monastery, a place of tranquility and contemplation. My decision and inquiry fortunately coincided with St. Christopher's need for a short-term Visiting Chaplain. Credentials, recommendations and availability meshed with fortuitous timing, and so I lived and worked at the Hospice from October 1 to December 30, 1974.

As Visiting Chaplain, I was accepted as a member of the top staff, befitting the stature of the clergy in the Church of England's scheme of things. I met almost daily with the admissions team and with nurses as they discussed their patients. I met weekly with administrators and programmers and became a member of two weekly discussion groups. I even sang in the staff choir. The coffee room, mid-mornings and afternoons was rife with animated and insightful conversations every day. I was free to chat with patients and their families as I wished. I was asked to conduct Sunday worship several times, and I conducted funeral services for two of the patients with whom I had worked closely.

Upon my return to the United States, I resigned my Kingston parish in order to devote my full time to the hospice movement at home. This meant liaison with Hospice, Inc., in New Haven (since renamed The Connecticut Hospice), the hospice prototype in the United States, involvement in the International Workshop on Death, Dying and Bereavement, leadership of numerous seminars and workshops on hospice care, and membership on the Board of Directors of the Society for the Right to Die, the "Living Will" group. But mostly it meant talking with people in Rhode Island about care of the dying and the grieving.

What surprised me was the number of people of a variety of backgrounds who had dreamed about establishing a hospice program in Rhode Island, but who almost unanimously felt they were alone in their dreams and hopes. Two groups have since emerged there: Thanatology Associates, Inc., which focuses primarily on counselling and education, and Hospice Care of Rhode Island, which aims at staff training and patient care.

This book, then, arises out of twenty-eight years of pastoral experience and five years of immersion in every phase of hospice care for the terminally ill. It is not a handbook of hospice organizations (there are now over two hundred such groups in the United States and Canada); nor is it an historical account of the hospice movement. Rather, this book attempts to define the hospice philosophy of caring for the terminally ill with the profound hope that it may be a resource to patients and their families, and, perhaps, even be a means of upgrading the health care industry's concern for the dying and the bereaved.

Introduction   xiii

Hospice Means Hope is also a way of saying thanks to many people: Dr. Cicely Saunders, for giving me a chance to learn at St. Christopher's; Bill Harvey, for including me in his dream project, The Home Care Association of Greater Providence; people like Charley Baldwin, Sid Cobb, Ray Gibson, Margaret MacColl Johnson, Irving Kronenberg, Marilyn Schlossberg, and the others who struggled to give Hospice Care of Rhode Island its birth; Marion Humphrey, Gene Knott, Claire Kowalski, Theresa Rando, Mike Scala, Barbara Wright and the cohorts in Thanatology Associates; Bev (R.N.) and Ralph (M.D.) Redding, sensitive friends and skillful practitioners of hospice arts. Finally, this book is a reality because of two groups of most supportive people: the Kingston Congregational Church, which made it possible for me to walk through the hospice door in the first place, and my present parish, the Pleasant Street Cogregational Church of Arlington, Massachusetts, colleagues in the endeavor to apply the hospice idea in our community.

To those who need it most,
HOSPICE MEANS HOPE

1

Hospice: a Definition

Far from being the quiet oasis for study and contemplation the word first suggested to me, a hospice is actually the arena for the most courageous activity imaginable. Originally, a hospice was a stopping place for weary travellers. During the Crusades, hospices were like Holiday Inns for devout and dedicated, but tired pilgrims. Whatever the origins and history, hospice today is an idea, a way of caring for the terminally ill, those weary travellers who are nearing the end of their earthly pilgrimage. The pioneer institution in the care of the terminally ill is appropriately named for St. Christopher, the patron saint of travellers.

Many people, at least the kindlier ones, have asked how a caregiver in a hospice can avoid becoming depressed. The answer is that he doesn't. The experience is a very heavy one. But the depressing factors are far outweighed by the inspirational. With rare exception, the hospice patients I have known have been concerned with living, not dying. Hubert Humphrey's advice to a fellow cancer sufferer "to live each day as though it were a gift" aptly defines the aim of most hospice patients. While it is most assuredly true that dying people can teach us much about dying, they can teach us even more about living. Their message is essentially, "Get your life priorities in order and then pursue them with a singleness of purpose."

Other people, less kindly disposed, wonder about my "morbid preoccupation with death." To that query I have two answers. First, I am persuaded that avoidance of the subject is far more unhealthy and harmful than an honest and positive confrontation. The second response is *Hospice Means Hope*.

Hospice: the Unique and the Universal

Each one of us lives a unique life, and each one of us dies in his or her own style. You inflict the grossest injustice upon others by imposing a supposed universal life-style upon the individual. Conversely, you express the highest respect for others by regarding their life-styles as unique.

Unfortunately, these simple precepts frequently crash into each other when applied to a dying individual. Who indeed can program another person's (or even his own) terminal trajectory? The way an individual dies is the way he dies. Nobody has ever died like that before and nobody ever will again. His emotional responses to the announcement of his pending death will, in all probability, be consistent with and reflect the way he has responded to other crises in his life. Consequently, he gains scant support from people who make assumptions about him. His defense mechanisms have enabled him to come this far, so it is cruel to destroy those defenses just because you happen to feel you know a better way for him to prepare for death.

Belief in the uniqueness of this individual is a cornerstone of the hospice philosophy. This belief, however, is apt to run afoul of two "higher authorities" in a health care system.

The first of these powerfully impersonal forces is institutional. Going to the hospital can be one of the most demeaning, coldly impersonal experiences in one's life. Very early in the game, probably when you are just sitting in the admissions office waiting for someone to collect your data, you become a cog in somebody else's machinery. It seems that every uniformed person in the place knows more about your condition than you do. Important decisions about you are made without your being consulted. And, most important of all, you soon learn the rule of conduct: well-behaved patients receive more attention and a pleasanter disposition than do ill-behaved patients. The more cantankerous you are, the more you grouse, the more you protest that nobody tells you anything, that you feel like a ping-pong ball, the more surly the response and, in time, the less frequent the attention.

This regrettable development is most predictable when a patient has the effrontery to be dying. More than one nurse has muttered, "I hope he doesn't die on my shift." After all, the medical world is geared to helping people get well. Those who don't get well pose a perplexing problem that is most easily handled by avoidance, by giving the dying person as wide a berth as possible. A cancer specialist underscored the point when he told a group of medical students: "Everybody knows that cancer patients get their medication fifteen minutes too late."

One sensitive doctor noticed that everyone on his hospital floor walked by the room of a certain dying patient. This behavior so puzzled the doctor that he asked a medical student to sit in the heavily sedated patient's room to monitor the visits he had in one daytime hour. The situation so intrigued the student that he remained an extra hour, then reported to the doctor that not one single person—not a member of the patient's family, not a member of the professional staff, not an orderly, not a housekeeper, not even a volunteer—had entered the patient's room in those two hours.

The second enemy of the individual's uniqueness comes in the form of general misinterpretations and misapplications of specific experience. Elizabeth Kübler-Ross has helped us learn valuable lessons from the dying. Her simple suggestion that if you want to find out what it is like to be dying you should listen to the dying apparently never occurred to health care professionals before. Her refreshing observation was like saying, "If you want to find out what it is like to be in prison, talk to a prisoner." It seems so obvious now.

From her extensive listening, Kübler-Ross has observed "five stages" in the dying process: denial, anger, bargaining, depression, and acceptance. These are emotional responses which she has observed and documented. Unfortunately for many dying people, well intentioned caregivers have interpreted and accepted those "five stages" as a necessary and unavoidable course which each patient must and will follow. These caregivers proceed to impose the "five stages" yardstick upon the terminally ill patient, and view their caring responsibility as that of leading, encouraging, even coaxing every patient to move along the course toward an inevitable acceptance of death.

Erroneous misinterpretation, faulty conclusion, zealous but misdirected good will . . . whatever. It is certainly not what Kübler-Ross had in mind when she reported her observations on the emotional responses of dying persons. Generalizing about a patient's needs and desires can be cruel. It is reminiscent of the mythological highwayman Procrustes who, after robbing his victims, placed them on a little iron bed and lopped off whatever parts of the body were hanging over the sides, so devoted was he to the virtue of absolute uniformity.

The true value of the "five stages," and it is considerable, is most fully realized when they are applied to the individual patient and his unique life and style. One minister, counselling the distraught wife of a man dying of cancer who had become very belligerent, pointed out to her that she was taking her husband's anger personally. "We are no longer in the dark about these things," he suggested. "Your husband's anger is such a perfectly normal reaction; but it is toward dying and not toward you. Chances are he will only feel guiltier and angrier if we are upset by his outbursts, or if we insist that he should not be angry." The minister's message was clear, person-centered and supportive of both the man and his wife: however he faces this crisis is the right way for him, and the best thing we can do for him is to support him by allowing him to have his way. Whether or not the dying person becomes depressed or a bargainer or an acceptor of his fate is not for us to determine. Only the individual can do that.

Hospice comes down solidly on the side of the unique, the personal. It is a stance that is concerned not with the treatment of a disease, but with the needs of a person. Hospice minimizes the importance of the institution or organization, and strives to make the patient and his family the center of concern.

I recall one cold, damp autumn day, the day Esther arrived at St. Christopher's Hospice. She was transferred quickly from the ambulance to the pre-warmed bed which had been wheeled to the door to meet her. Her bed was moved directly to her place on the ward. The doctor greeted her there, offered her and her husband a cup of tea, introduced them to the other patients on the ward, suggested they relax together for a while, and promised that someone from the office would be around shortly to sit down and fill out the simple but necessary forms. Esther was treated as a person, not as an additional cog in a health care system's machinery.

Another St. Christopher's patient, William Franklin, told me that he was in and out of so many hospitals and offices and clinics that he didn't care what happened to him anymore: "It was always wait . . . get up and get this paper . . . sit down and wait . . . talk to this secretary . . . go to that office. It burnt me flippin' wick, I tell ya! Then I found out I was going to be sent to the 'hospick.' And you know what happened? When I got here, Matron met me at the door and said, 'Hello, Mr. Franklin, welcome to St. Christopher's.' Nobody ever treated me like that since I've been sick. I'm lucky to be here." At St. Christopher's, Mr. Franklin was treated with the respect a living human being deserves.

Hospice: Quality of Life

"Death with Dignity," I had thought, was one of those emotionally triggered cliches to which speakers run when they have not examined their subject very thoroughly or when somebody asks them a too thoughtful question. So too, I surmised, "Quality of Life" was an empty banality. Exposure to hospice care, however, raised simple questions which, I am now embarrassed to admit, I had not previously considered: "What do you mean by dignity?" and "Who decides what kind of quality?" An answer to the second question helps to answer the first. The patient and his family determine what is meaningful for them, what constitutes quality of life. Hospice caregivers believe strongly in the family's right to determine how they will handle their problems and live out their lives. Undebatable? Obvious? So it would seem.

However, the initiative is frequently taken away from patients and their families by a health care industry that, in our day, has assumed and presumed almost divine authority over human lives. The Quinlan case is an example. It is, however, *only* an example, for there are countless numbers of persons, declared terminally ill, for whom the Quinlans' helplessness is something of a prototype. Their name is Legion, which may account in part for the notoriety of the Quinlan case. Once Karen Quinlan's life-sustaining machinery was plugged in, it seemed that every known source of authority got into the act: judges, doctors, lawyers, clergy, psychiatrists, et al. Everyone wanted to help decide on matters of "quality" and "dignity."

Hospice people feel that the families, not the professional helpers, must play the major role in life and death decisions. The families must decide the type and the amount of quality they will seek for their loved ones and for themselves. Hospice caregivers support the family in their final determination of what "dignity" is for them, and the way they maintain this support makes "Quality of Life" a beautiful reality and "Death with Dignity" far more than a cliche.

No Machine, No Plugs

Another cornerstone of the hospice movement philosophy is the belief that a good life deserves a good death. When no further treatment of the illness is prescribed, hospice does everything possible to keep the patient comfortable and to let him die naturally when his time comes. There is no painful hanging on, no aching clinging to a life that is ending. Surgical procedures are followed only to decrease pain and to increase comfort. If, for example, a tracheotomy would aid a patient's breathing, the operation would be performed without hesitation. Hospice care is guided by the belief that a cup of tea, patiently and lovingly fed on a patient's last day, means more to that patient than any and all death-prolonging machinery.

Time Within Time

The primary concern of hospice, what its care is all about, is simply treating patients as living human beings and not as people who are about to die. These people, enduring the withdrawal of their very existence, are striving to live as fully as they can before they die.

The ancient Greeks could describe this search for quality in life far better than we can because when it was necessary they used more than one word to denote different experiences. They had, for example, four words for our one word "love." They used two words for "time" because they understood time to have two meanings. One of these words, *chronos,* is the base for all our time definitions—chronology, chronicle, chronic, and a good many more. *Chronos* is objective time. It is the dispassionate ticking of the clock, the "three-score-and-ten" years of life expectancy. Our medical research and prevention and regimens and surgical procedures are aimed at one thing and one thing only—to extend everybody's chronological age.

Early in 1978, NBC ran a two-hour TV special on health care in this country which unknowingly demonstrated the health care industry's overriding concern with *chronos.* They devoted roughly an hour and a quarter to preventing, curing, healing and paying for preventing, curing, and healing. They devoted half an hour to research and speculation on methods which might radically increase life-expectancy. They spent less than ten minutes on sensitive care of the dying. Clearly, our health care system majors in longevity, in *chronos.*

Our language has no derivatives from the other Greek word for time—*kairos. Kairos* is qualitative time, subjective time, time unique to each person. *Kairos* involves accomplishment, fulfillment, emotion, richness. It is the dynamic that makes an hour spent with a dear friend seem only a single minute, and twenty-minute sermons (some of them at least) seem twenty hours long. "Sportin' Life" in *Porgy and Bess* knew the difference between *chronos* and *kairos* when he sang, "Methuselah lived nine-hundred years . . . but who calls that livin' . . . when no gal will give in to no man what's nine-hundred years?"

Hospice care assists people in making whatever time is left to them qualitative time—in filling whatever *chronos* remains with as much *kairos* as possible—with the patients and their families deciding what is *kairos* to them.

Formula for Creative Caring

People have to find their own "quality" and "dignity," to be sure. But their quest becomes more fruitful with a little help from their friends. Friends can help in this search for "quality" and "dignity" by applying a little formula first posited by Frank Laubach, the renowned Christian missionary and originator of the "each one teach one" literacy program in underdeveloped areas of the world. Laubach suggests that you find out what a person is proud of and praise him for it; find out what a person needs and give it to him. It is a simple formula, but in order to discover what a person needs and what he is proud of, you have to listen—and when you listen, you have to hear.

Comfort and Company

Two of the most frequently expressed fears of dying people are the fear of an agonizing, painful death and the fear of being forgotten, uncared about, ignored, left alone. These fears are expressed so often, they are practically axiomatic. Hospice care helps mitigate these fears.

Evelyn was one of a handful of motor-neuron patients at St. Christopher's. The dying process was, therefore, a good deal more protracted for her than for her fellow patients, most of whom were victims of cancer. She had been in her four-bed ward for about a year; the other three beds were occupied by cancer patients. She had seen almost seventy people—seventy friends—die. Yet, she was one of the most chipper people in the building, staff included. I once asked her how she kept from being depressed. Without batting an eye, and with her infectious smile, she replied simply, "I have never seen anyone die alone, and I have never seen anyone die in agony at St. Christopher's." She paused a moment, then added, "Depressed? How could I be when I'm in the best place for me in all the world?" Amazingly enough, Evelyn was reinforced every time one of her ward mates died, and she herself had become a most reassuring source of comfort and company for other patients in the hospice.

Listening and Hearing

Even in the altered environment hospice offers, you can't be very helpful to a terminally ill person if he doesn't trust you. The question of whether he trusts you or not is almost entirely up to you. If you present yourself as a listener, then you had better listen or risk not being taken seriously. A patient discovers very early whether you are a talker or a listener. And the terminally ill, with little to gain by playing games with you, can be refreshingly candid—and sometimes painfully helpful.

I went to St. Christopher's determined to learn some things about the end of life from people who were actually experiencing it. I was there to listen. That was my promise, implied if not announced, as Visiting Chaplain. Within a month I felt confident that I was listening well. But one unforgettable day, a woman named Myrtle taught me that "once a talker, always a talker."

Myrtle and I had some good talks together during the early part of my stay at St. Christopher's; we were friends. In her last days, Myrtle was generally comatose. I would stop in to see her a couple of times a day. I would say, "Hello, Myrtle," then I would touch her arm or her forehead. She would not speak— she seemed not to have enough strength for speech—but once in a while she would open her jaundiced eyes and manage a faint smile. One day upon arriving, I noticed that she was sleeping. I decided to visit the other patients on the floor first, then work my way back up to Myrtle's bed. When I finally got to Myrtle, I touched her, said hello, and saw her eyes open. Then she struggled to speak. "My goodness but your voice must be sore," she said, "I've heard you coming all the way down the hall." It was the last time she ever spoke to me. Those may have been her last words to anybody, for she died the next day. I know I will never stop hearing those words. Myrtle shook me up, and I hope she made me a better listener.

Listening, however, does not mean merely hearing and understanding the other person. It also means responding to what you hear, and responding spontaneously. Martha taught me that.

Martha was a woman of many honest moods. One morning when I entered St. Christopher's she was crying quietly. She motioned me to sit down. She wiped her eyes, blew her nose, and held up a note she had just received in the day's mail. One of her dearest friends had just died. I told her I was sorry and asked her to tell me about her friend and about their friendship. She did, at some length.

When I went to see her next morning, she greeted me with, "I've written something I would like to share with you." She handed me a card on which she had scrawled these words: "When someone dear dies, you just feel your own sense of loss. Your greatest fear is that there will be no one left to love you. Deep in all of us lies a certain fear that no one values us, wants us, needs us." I said that was a very touching tribute to their friendship, and I thanked her for sharing those deep thoughts with me. Then I left.

Half-way down the hall the truth hit me. Martha's words were not a soliloquy on the death of a friend. She was asking me, "Am I of any value to you?" I had missed an opportunity for spontaneity. But only for the moment it took me to race back to her room to tell her "Yes!"

2

Hospice: Health Care Bridge

Hospice care of the terminally ill began because of a critical lack in health care services. Noticeable gaps exist (1) between treating the disease and treating the person, (2) between technological research and psycho-social support, and (3) between the general denial of the fact of death in our society and the acceptance of death by those who face it.

Some time ago I participated in a seminar of medical students who were in the last term of their last year of medical school and had elected a course in community health. My experience with this particular group underscored the medical community's tendency to treat the disease but to ignore the person.

The professor had designed the course to enable the students to discover the needs of cancer patients and to ascertain how the resources of the community were being used to meet those needs. My job was to assign each of the ten students one terminally ill cancer patient. The students would center their attention on their patients, assess the patients' needs and suggest ways of bringing community resources to bear on their behalf. At the first meeting of the students, one week into the project, one of the students requested another assignment. "My patient is being well taken care of," he said. "He's getting all the medical care he needs. There's nothing more I can give him, so I'd like another one." The professor then asked the salient question: "What about the patient's non-medical needs?" The student replied, "What do you mean, 'non-medical' needs?" Our health care system encourages the almost complete compartmentalization of the patient, with medical people focussing almost exclusively on the physical body.

The gap between technological research and psycho-social support was made sadly apparent to a friend of mine at the age of thirty-two. He had broken his arm playing hockey. His doctor said the x-rays showed an unusual condition and suggested he go to Sloane-Kettering in New York, a Mecca for cancer patients in the United States. The doctor avoided any mention of possible malignancy and thus avoided further conversation with the patient about his condition.

At Sloan-Kettering, the specialists examined my friend and announced that they would have to amputate his left arm in order to save his life. Nobody asked him how he felt about the alternatives. No one asked him for any input in the decision process. The decision had simply already been made for him by other people. Since the message was blatantly clear, and since he really had no choice, he agreed to the amputation.

He was alone in a private room. That first night, nobody talked with him about his situation. Nobody asked how he felt, what he feared, what his hopes and expectations were, what his family thought—nothing. Various staff persons came in, of course, to perform their duties: they took his temperature, recorded his blood pressure, felt his pulse. But nobody talked with him personally. "Once," he later told me, "a resident doctor and a nurse were in my room at the same time, but all the while they were going about their business, he was trying to make a date with her."

Then they brought him his first meal—roast beef. They wheeled it in, and then walked out again. He sat there with his broken arm in a sling, but nobody had bothered to cut his meat for him.

When my friend speaks of his experience at Sloan-Kettering (and what happened to him in that oncological Shangri-la is typical of the experiences of many cancer patients in most hospitals today) he says, "They removed my left arm; I know they saved my life. But they raped my soul."

The health care industry in this country spends millions of dollars to advance medical technology, millions of dollars on education, research, prevention, cure and rehabilitation for the two-thirds of the people who have cancer and who are going to get well—or who at least have their life span extended a bit. But health care organizations, even such organizations as the American Cancer Society, spend very little on the other third, those cancer patients who are going to die of the disease. The medical community, like the society of which it is part, has difficulty accepting the fact of death.

A Boston area physician called the chairman of a community group which had begun planning a program for local hospice services. The physician asked if there were anyone in the group who might visit with one of his patients who was at home in an advanced stage of cancer. The patient also needed someone to transport him to the physician's office for periodic monitoring of his condition; ambulance costs were prohibitive for the patient.

"We can find someone to visit him," replied the chairman. "But have you tried the Cancer Society for transportation help?"

The doctor paused, then said, "The Cancer Society doesn't help people. They just raise money."

It is, perhaps, unfair to single out the American Cancer Society, for it spends its money the way the federal and state health care programs do and the way third-party reimbursers (Blue Cross, et al) do—to help those who can make it through the ordeal. Who, indeed, would begrudge the money spent on research and treatment?

However, hospice people ask, "What about the one-third who die from cancer?" The patients themselves ask the question more poignantly: "What are you doing to help us die with dignity?" And the reply from the American Cancer Society, as well as from the entire health care system, has been "Nothing. Sorry." When a person cannot recover, an entire multi-million dollar health care system stops supporting him.

The Bridge Builder

The health care community is concerned with prevention, treatment, rehabilitation and cure, and we all thank God for their concerns. But it has more often than not indifferently turned its back upon people for whom there is no more treatment, no more cure, no more rehabilitation.

A major problem facing many cancer patients, one that has been largely ignored or, at best, only casually dealt with by the medical profession, is the all-consuming agony of chronic pain. Chronic pain—unlike acute pain that is temporary and which, in time, abates and disappears—not only does not go away; it increases until the sufferer dies.

Those who care personally about patients trapped by chronic pain have long been raising questions about the seemingly unsolvable mystery: Why should people have to suffer like this? Why do they have to be rendered vegetables in order to be made barely comfortable? Such questions, so long unaddressed medically, have testified to the enormous chasm that has separated the terminally ill patient from the most sophisticated health care industry in history. Consequently, the overarching purpose of the hospice movement is to bridge that chasm, to relieve the suffering of the dying and to support them and their families in every way possible.

One might accurately state that hospice care began when humans first responded to the needs of their fellow humans, that caring is as old as the human race. But as societies and technologies became more complex, sophisticated caring systems grew apace. To point, then, to any one place, or to any one person or group and say "Lo, hospice began here," or "It all started with them" would do a gross injustice to the host of forerunners to what today is called "hospice." Nevertheless, most hospice people agree that the modern movement began in Great Britain. And many point to the work of the Irish Sisters of Charity at St. Joseph's Hospice, London, as having built a bridge between the needs of terminally ill cancer patients and the medical profession.

For a long time, the Sisters of Charity at St. Joseph's Hospice have been concerned about the problems of chronic pain and have sought ways of keeping patients comfortable yet lucid. In the mid-1950's, the St. Joseph's staff welcomed Dr. Cicely Saunders as an ally in the development of pain control techniques. Dr. Saunders would later become the founding spirit of St. Christopher's Hospice, London, and be recognized widely as the individual most responsible for the beginnings of the hospice movement in the United States.

There was more to the St. Joseph's experience for Dr. Saunders than the exciting and gratifying exploration of pain control regimes. Forty-five patients were dying of cancer. But they were alert. They were serene. None of them seemed to be in pain. Some even had remissions, enabling them to go home for awhile. Depression was a rarity rather than the norm. How did it all happen? Why were those patients so free of the anxieties and pain which one usually associates with terminal cancer? The answer to those questions is what constitutes "hospice."

At the very heart of hospice care is a community of caregivers who work at and live in an aura of harmony and mutual respect. Their spirit can only be described, finally, as religious, in the deepest sense and in the widest, non-sectarian application of the word. Religious devotion to their patients and colleagues is the hallmark of hospice caregivers.

Adaptable Care Package

On April 10, 1967, the new St. Christopher's Hospice, located in the Sydenham section of London, opened its doors. Dr. Cicely Saunders, the Medical Director, and four other staff persons were on hand. The first patient was admitted to the fifty-four bed facility three months later. Each of the three floors has been arranged to accommodate patients in four to six bed wards. A few private rooms are maintained for special-needs patients.

With few exceptions, the patients at St. Christopher's are dying of cancer. They are admitted if they have a chronic pain problem, if no further treatment of their cancer is suggested, if they have a short prognosis (in days and weeks, not months and years), and if they cannot be supported at home. The mean age is forty-nine. The average stay for cancer patients is thirteen days. Despite the number of deaths, bed occupancy stays close to ninety percent. The list of applicants to St. Christopher's is substantial, and those waiting for admission are asked to be prepared to come to the Hospice as soon as possible after they are called.

Since opening its doors in 1967, St. Christopher's has

maintained a home care program which is designed to offer twenty-four-hour-a-day, seven-day-a-week support of the patient and the family. After chronic pain and terminality, two criteria for home care support stand out: the patient must want to stay at home and the family must want him there. Most St. Christopher's admissions are placed in the home care program, and many admissions to the inpatient facility come from this program. But whether to inpatient facility or to home care, when a patient is accepted by St. Christopher's he is assured of continuing support and care. When the nursing burden becomes too taxing at home, a bed for the patients will be found in the inpatient facility. Should patients be able to go home again for a while, as many do, they are assured that a bed will always be available to them when they need it.

It is important to remember that the hospice philosophy of caring is not limited to a free-standing inpatient facility. While such a facility is ideal, it is also extremely costly to the point of being prohibitive. And the final justification of the hospice movement is not whether a brand new medical institution has been introduced into our society, but whether hospice has enabled existing health care institutions to take dying patients seriously and to upgrade the quality of their care. Hospice groups in this country, therefore, begin by spreading the word as best they can and in the ways that are immediately open to them. Presumably, each group dreams of establishing an inpatient facility, but the dream does not prevent them from starting where they are, or, more accurately, where the opportunities are.

The Connecticut Hospice in New Haven conducted a hospice home care program for over seven years before actually breaking ground for their new inpatient facility. Palliative Care units have been conducting pilot programs for the control of chronic pain in such places as St. Luke's Hospital in New York, Methodist Hospital in Indianapolis and Royal Victoria Hospital in Montreal. Some groups have begun by training volunteers for a local Visiting Nurse Association, or by conducting workshops and seminars for professional health care people, or by introducing chronic pain control techniques to local cancer specialists, or by offering counselling support for dying patients and their families and for the widowed. Other groups are designing hospice programs in cooperation with the administrators of hospitals and nursing residences. Some groups are formally organized and incorporated; others are loose affiliations, but no less influential in their local communities. The growing inclusion of hospice ideas into medical and nursing school curricula is one of the movement's brightest hopes.

The point is, hospice is a philosophy, a way of caring for the terminally ill for whom all restorative and curative treatments have been abandoned. Hospice is a kind of "care package," and the package includes only four essential elements:

(1) Control of chronic pain
(2) Realism about death
(3) The "family" as the primary unit of caring
(4) Staff support systems

Whatever else may be added along the way, a hospice program can be identified by these four characteristics.

3

Control of Chronic Pain

"You don't really care about a patient if you don't care about his pain." This is the bluntly axiomatic point of origin for the hospice care of the terminally ill. A dying person has little concern for the "quality of life" if he is perpetually plagued with excruciating pain. One evening after I had spoken about the need to control chronic pain, a young man told me of his grandfather who had endured unbelievable suffering for seven months as he was dying of cancer. In the last two months, he had only enough energy to speak to members of his family for perhaps two minutes at a time at wide intervals. The rest of the dying man's time was spent fighting the pain.

The hospice movement's major contribution to the field of medicine is the successful introduction of a program of effective control of chronic pain. The control regimen involves four essential parts:
 (1) the right analgesic
 (2) in the least amount necessary
 (3) at the right time
 (4) in the most effective manner.

The Right Analgesic

When a person is dying, you worry about his pain. You do not worry about possible addiction. If you really care about his pain, you will employ any agent or procedure that will give him relief. Even if surgery is no longer recommended for treatment, it might be employed to lessen the patient's pain, as in the severing of a nerve, for instance.

The hospice movement has introduced a palliative formula based on a mixture once used in the old Brompton Hospital in London. It is appropriately dubbed "Brompton's Mixture," though pharamaceutical variations result in a variety of appellations such as "Brompton's Cocktail" and "Pain Cocktail." The mixture originally included heroin, cocaine, alcohol and an elixir. While it is generally agreed that heroin is the most effective known pain reliever (and there is, at last, movement afoot in this country to legalize its use for analgesic purposes), morphine is a highly acceptable substitute in "Brompton's Mixture."

At St. Christopher's, Robert Twycross conducted an extensive six-month testing of the effectiveness of both heroin—which may be legally employed in England—and morphine, and he found that both are effective and acceptable in the control of chronic pain. Ongoing palliative care experiments are substituting a variety of other drugs in the search for more effective treatment of pain.

The assortment of ingredients in "Brompton's Mixture" suggests that chronic pain is caused by a number of things, and is not just physiological. Anxiety about pain can heighten pain, depression can increase pain, and so on. "Brompton's Mixture" is designed to alleviate all levels and kinds of pain.

In the Least Amount Necessary

In this country the usual method for treating chronic pain is to have the patient take pills and receive injections that are more than sufficient to control pain. This results in the overkill of pain. The body builds up a tolerance to the medication, so more and more painkillers are necessary. In time, relief comes only from strong narcotics injected p.r.n. (as needed). After a while, no amount of drugs within the parameters determined by the doctor—who may fear that increased doses will kill the patient—can ease the pain. The only hope is that the injections will knock the patient out for some time. This means that every waking moment is pain-filled, and every pain-free moment is lived in unconsciousness.

The hospice regimen requires not the most, but the least

amount of analgesics necessary to control pain. The two-fold aim of the regimen is to keep the patient comfortable and to enable him to remain lucid and coherent. The patient needs to know that the pain will not recur and that he will no longer have to play games with the nurses, games such as asking for the medication before he needs it because he knows the nurse will be slow in giving it to him. He needs to be freed from the fear that his pain will return.

In the Most Effective Manner

"Brompton's" is administered orally so that the relief will be even and level. Relief from injected medications is more like peaks and valleys. Oral medication also eliminates two possibly demeaning addictions: reliance upon a needle (not a drug, but a needle) and reliance upon the nurse who gives the injection that brings desperately longed-for relief. An additional advantage of oral medication is that tolerance builds more slowly than it does with injections. Consequently, with a much slower increase in dosage strength and a pattern of administering the least amount necessary, patients require less drugs than are ordinarily required for an overkill of the pain.

At the Right Time

The right time is before the pain hits! Medication given in anticipation of pain enables the patient to be free from pain and free from the fear of pain. It is a beautiful day when a person who has not had a pain-free minute for six months finds himself comfortable. This does, however, suggest one of the problems sometimes encountered in using "Brompton's."

Chronic pain can frequently be brought under control within twenty-four hours by regular medication every three to four hours, before the pain recurs. Many a patient has felt so good, at times bordering on elated disbelief, that he sees no reason for continuing medication. After all, when one is feeling so good, why should one take medication? If there is no pain, why take something for the relief of pain? Further, the patient may also see his comfort as an opportunity to minimize the chances of drug addiction for him. In some instances, a good deal of persuasion is required to convince the patient that he will not become a drug addict using "Brompton's" and that he must continue to take the medication on schedule if he is to continue the comfort. The doctor will experiment with a weaker dosage (the *least* amount necessary), but the patient must take the "Brompton's" on schedule.

With all the persuasion in the world, however, some patients feel so good that they plot to avoid taking their medicine. And they discover, much to their discomfort, that the counselling voices were absolutely right. The pain returns, possibly requiring heavier medication to again bring the pain under control. Amazingly, or perhaps not so amazingly, some patients run through this process again and again. And each time they relearn the essential lesson: You must take the medication religiously on schedule, before the pain hits! You know that chronic pain, unlike acute pain, will recur. To get on top of it, you must take medication in anticipation, as a prophylaxis.

Possible Problems and Complications

In the treatment of acute pain, nurses may be reluctant to awaken a sleeping patient in order to give him his medication. They may feel that since he hasn't asked for it that he doesn't need it, that he is comfortable and that they should not disturb him. The ugly truth about chronic pain, however, is that it will recur if it is ignored. The patient must, therefore, be awakened and the medication given on schedule to insure continuing, uninterrupted comfort.

Another problem arises with doctors who, upon hearing about "Brompton's Mixture," throw up their hands and say, in effect, "You'll never be able to get the druggist to fill that prescription." The truth of the matter is that pharmacists are generally extremely cooperative. Once you explain the program to them, once you tell them this medication can relieve chronic pain and yet enable the patient to remain lucid, they are more than eager to cooperate. The suggestion that pharmacists will not cooperate because they do not want supplies of cocaine on hand does not stand up in actual experience.

Some side effects, such as nausea, which is typical in the administration of some narcotics, do require special treatment. But there is a wealth of information to be gleaned from hospice groups with extensive experience on how to cope with these side effects. For example, syrup of prochlorperazine, or compazine, can be added for nausea and usually synergizes the effect of "Brompton's Mixture." Other hospice physicians order the compazine to be taken a half hour before the "Brompton's."

One doctor, using "Brompton's" for the first time, stated that although it relieved the pain, it seemed to make patients as drowsy as they were with other medications. It turned out that the doctor instructed the patients to take supplementary doses as needed (p.r.n. again). This instruction explained the drowsiness. If the dosage does not control the pain, the next dosage should be stronger (the least amount to *control* the pain) and continued on the regular regimen. But supplementary doses limit the overall effect.

Another doctor's patients sometimes became disoriented when starting on the "Brompton's" regimen. At the slightest hint of disorientation, this doctor tended to abandon the formula, concluding that this particular patient could not be helped by it. Hospice physicians, with a confidence in the formula that is based upon broad experience, counter this procedure with a plea to give the new medication a bit more time to prove its effectiveness. They suggest allowing as much as seventy-two hours for the patient to adjust, and for the attending physician to make minor changes in order to determine the "right" dosage for the patient. With a bit more patience and with closer monitoring of the patient's responses, the initial period of disorientation should pass.

The use of the hospice formula for the control of chronic pain obviously requires a good deal of monitoring, or titration. This is most necessary within the first twenty-four hours, and then in the first several days. The purpose of titration is to make sure that the patient's pain is under control and that he is not being over-dosed.

One of the most positive aspects in the entire regimen is the degree of control which the patient has over the entire medicating process. It is the patient—and only the patient—who can tell you if he is in pain, and in how much pain. Doctors and nurses, therefore, need to ask the patient regularly if he is in pain. The information must then be shared, and modifications ordered accordingly by the doctor.

Cost

Enough "Brompton's Mixture" to control a person's pain for one week costs less than $10.

Effectiveness

One must experience the "before and after" effect of "Brompton's Mixture" in order to begin to truly appreciate what a precious contribution it is to medicine. I recall one young woman with lung cancer who was admitted to St. Christopher's; every breath she had taken for the past four months had been labored and painful. Within one day the pain was gone, the breathing eased. She was truly elated when she said, "I really believed I would never again draw an easy breath!"

St. Christopher's has been "a place for weary travelers" to over five thousand patients now. With few exceptions, they all had chronic pain problems. Other hospices and Palliative Care programs have treated equally as many, if not many more, chronic pain patients. The results are astonishing: from ninety to ninety-six percent of the patients had their pain brought under control without experiencing either euphoria or loss of consciousness! That means that all the energy which had been expended in combatting severe pain could now be reinvested in making the days count for as much as possible, in adding *kairos* to the remaining days.

In recent years, other hospice programs have been experimenting with different drugs and have found many of them effective substitutes for "Brompton's." What is becoming clearer every day is that the actual drugs used are not as important in pain control format as the manner in which they are employed. The hospice formula for the control of chronic pain remains all important: the right analgesic, in the least amount necessary, in the most effective manner, at the right time.

Amazing and often times miraculous things have happened to some patients who, with their agonizing pain a thing of the past, are supported with intelligent and tender loving care. Top staff people at St. Christopher's estimate that as high as six percent of their patients, people who had a very short prognosis when they arrived, actually enjoy a period of remission. No one knows how or why, and no one really cares how or why. They only know that once in a while it happens. And when it happens, it is a story that bears repeating. Like the story of Mary.

Mary was a thirty-five year old nurse, a single woman who lived at home with her parents. She was an only child. When doctors discovered a malignant brain tumor, Mary's parents became over-protective and, at the same time, over-critical. They had always controlled Mary's life rather rigorously, and their tendency to control blossomed unattractively as Mary's condition worsened. Both Mary's physical condition and her home surroundings were liabilities to her.

When she was admitted to St. Christopher's, the doctors gave her about ten days to live. She had lost her speech. She was heavily sedated and was consequently rarely awake. She lay immobile on her bed. Within twelve hours after going on "Brompton's Mixture," however, Mary's pain was gone, and in two weeks she was actually sitting on the edge of her bed. As her condition improved, she began going home for weekends. The hospice social worker helped Mary's parents become more creatively supportive of their daughter. In time, those weekends became increasingly delightful for all three people, as well as for the children of some cousins who now found "Aunt Mary" a far nicer person than they had ever remembered.

When I began my stay at St. Christopher's, Mary had been there an entire year. She now spent most of her day in a wheelchair. She was learning to knit. She had regained her speech to a great degree. She was a remarkably cheerful lady. She had no pain, and she did not look like a person with only a few weeks to live. One afternoon, eighteen staff people—doctors, nurses, administrators, social workers, physical therapist, psychiatrist, chaplain, porters, anyone who had a bit of insight into Mary—gathered to discuss Mary's future. They all agreed she should go someplace where she could participate in a more aggressively therapeutic program. The doctor said that Mary's prognosis was now at least ten years. The group came up with some possible choices for Mary, and the doctor agreed to present these possibilities to her for her decision.

Now, the St. Christopher's staff did nothing for Mary except control her pain, express support for her family and love her as a person. Mary found new energy for living because hospice people cared creatively. They began with concern for her pain. And that is where hospice care must always begin.

4

Realism About Death

The hospice movement is waging heroic battle against some formidable mythological dragons. One such myth concerns realism and hope.

In our society's discomfort with the subject of death, manifested glaringly by our preoccupation with cure and longevity and by funeral practices that attempt to conceal the reality of death, we have come to believe that if a person knows he is dying he will lose all hope. Keep the patient looking ahead, we say, and he will hang on. Tell him he is going to die, and he will give up. Keep him looking ahead and he won't be depressed by his lot today. It's the old carrot-before-the-donkey ploy.

The premise, or course, is sound. A person needs meaning to want to live; and without meaning, the motivation to live evaporates. The fallacy in the argument is that longevity is not the all-important incentive in life. While the drive for survival is crucial, it is not, finally, the most potent force for those who face death. Near the end, the most precious goal is quality. The question "What can I do to make this day count the most?" is paramount to the dying. "How long can I live?" is of far less consequence.

Hospice people are saying forthrightly that superficial and undue emphasis upon longevity actually impedes the patient's quest for meaning, and that supportive honesty is the best defense against hopelessness and despair. To be sure, a dying person will in all probability suffer waves of despair. But a cover-up does little more than prolong that despair. Thus, the hospice stance toward realism concerning death is far more than a mere suggestion or theory. It is a frontal attack on a dragon. And experience corroborates the claim and bolsters the attack.

Creative caring begins with control of pain. But pain control is not enough, in itself, to assure quality of life. The hospice experience testifies to the need for strong psycho-social support for the patient and his family, and asserts that an air of realism and truthfulness is one of the basic elements in that support. Within the framework of openness and caring, patients are able to be more creative, more relaxed, and of all things, even more joyful and more appreciative of each day.

Two Different Languages

Subterfuge, half-truths and blatant lies create confusion for the patient, and confusion is a major nemesis for the dying person. Part of the confusion is due to honest miscommunication. Doctors seem to talk a different language—"medicalese." How does the patient know that "You have a short prognosis" means "You are going to die soon"? At the same time, the patient and his family may be so caught up in the emotion of the situation that they wouldn't hear the doctor if he told them the truth in plain layman's English.

A friend told me about her father who had suddenly collapsed one day. They rushed him to the hospital, then waited the long eons one endures in anxious anticipation of some word from the examining doctor. When the doctor arrived, he very carefully tried to explain to the man's wife, daughter and son-in-law that he had had a stroke. The doctor went on to tell them what they could expect. When the three of them got home, each had quite a different notion of what the doctor had said, and all were baffled by what they felt had not been said. Out of that experience my friend expressed the wish that hospitals might provide interpreters who, as often as repetition was necessary, could help families understand what the professional health-care people were saying.

Hospice people fully realize the need for clarification of medical terminology to the patient and his family. This awareness is one of their hallmarks. They assume nothing.

They constantly double and triple check to make sure that the patient and his family are getting straight answers to their questions and that they understand the answers. Further realizing that patients frequently block out answers to protect themselves, support-givers exercise extreme patience during this process.

"Bermuda in the Spring"

The main confusion, however, stems not so much from lack of communication as from conflicting information. More than employing the simple defense mechanism of not hearing, most patients hear clearly what is said. And more. There seems little doubt these days that a patient knows what is going on in his body. Covering up the truth only compounds his confusion. It also saps his energy, forcing him to cover up in order to protect others who, he thinks, do not know. George Riley was one such patient.

At the age of sixty, George Riley was operated on for cancer of the esophagus. The surgeon, finding the malignancy widespread, removed as much of the growth as he could, but he knew that Riley's condition was fatal. He told George's wife, Hattie, what he had found, but strongly warned her against saying anything to her husband; he feared the knowledge of his condition would radically worsen George's physical state, cause deep depression and hasten his death.

When George came out of the recovery room, he was immediately aware of sharp pains all the way from his stomach around his side and up his back. He asked the surgeon why he had cut so far. The doctor replied it was standard operating procedure. When George later complained of excruciating pain deep in the area of the incision near his left shoulder blade, the doctor told him that it was post-operative pain, acute pain, and that it was normal. The doctor persisted in that answer for eight months, even though the pain kept increasing not abating.

George later told a confidant that he knew the truth of the matter as soon as he was aware of the extensive surgery, and that his strong suspicions were confirmed when the pain not only did not subside, but actually increased. Until the truth was out for all to see, George was tormented by conflicting "truths," and was desperately alone in his belief that his wife did not know. George's desperation was matched by her frustration over having to keep the painful secret from him.

Professional caregivers are powerful figures to the dying person, and, more than any others, are at fault in fanning the spark of false hopes for the patient. Most of the time, the deception is intentional. When a nurse cheerfully says, "You'll be in Bermuda in the Spring"—not because she believes it, but because she thinks it best for the patient that she be "hopeful"—it sets into motion a whole scenario of fantasy, most gladly indulged in, which clashes brutally with what the patient strongly knows to be the truth. Confusion! False hopes! Opportunities of today by-passed for tomorrow's mirage! It takes only one well-intentioned but misguided professional caregiver to raise in the patient the suspicion, the hope, that just possibly nobody knows for sure after all if he will live or die.

Nor are the patient's friends much help, although their desire to protect may be the more forgiveable, or at least the more understandable. Wanting to help, but feeling terribly frustrated, helpless and awkward, the friends may unwittingly contribute to the hodge-podge of emotion by suggesting, "You'll surely be going home soon." And inwardly the patient responds with, "Well, why can't I go home?" He knows why, of course, but it's worth a try.

Professional Projection

An increasingly accepted hypothesis in the current study of death and dying is that people who have not faced their own mortality realistically cannot be expected to help others face theirs creatively. In fact, the more threatening death is to us, the more protective we shall probably be to avoid the truth of the matter. A number of studies on the subject indicate that health care professionals are more uptight about fatal illness than are the laity. Doctors appear to be the most reluctant to face the reality of their own illness. It is not just a matter of their being trained to cure, and that, as one cancer specialist told me, every failure to cure is a defeat that cuts doctors very deeply. Many doctors, cancer specialists included, simply would not want to be told if they were terminally ill.

The surgeon who operated on George Riley was being besieged by George's wife, who said the doctor was avoiding her. She caught up with him late one afternoon in the hospital parking lot, and asked him why he was misleading George about his illness and giving him false hope. The doctor replied, "My dear, you must get ahold of yourself or you'll go to pieces. You are smoking too much and you are drinking too much. You're on your way to becoming an alcoholic and a psychotic."

Hattie was momentarily stunned. But she managed to fire a final salvo at the departing doctor. "Doctor," she said, "I hope that when you are as sick as George, your wife will get more support and understanding from her doctor than you are giving me."

The doctor spun around and said, "Mrs. Riley, my wife will never be in your position. If I ever find out that I've got terminal cancer, I'll blow my brains out!" In that moment, Hattie knew why her doctor had not been more helpful and supportive. The threat of terminal illness was too overwhelming for him to face.

To Tell Or Not to Tell

This is the perennial question. To hospice people, however, it is the wrong question. The issue is not whether to tell, but what, and how and when to tell. Hospice people believe that every patient has the right to know what is happening to his life, and that every answer given to every question must be the truth. It need not be the whole truth, but it must be the truth. And the truth must be spoken within the framework of caring. Bluntness is no virtue. Blatant honesty is a false god. Cold facts can hurt badly, sometimes irreparably.

I once heard a priest, a member of a panel, talk about his own cancer. He had discovered a lump and went to see his doctor. The doctor sent him to a clinic for a biopsy. Three days later, the doctor called and said, "Father Smith, you've got cancer. Come in and see me." Then he hung up. That's a pretty tough way to learn you have cancer. It makes for a difficult day. Father Smith certainly wanted the information, he said, but he needed it under less devastating circumstances.

The hospice movement champions a compassionate realism concerning the dying process. And a compassionate yet realistic doctor is perhaps the greatest asset a dying person can have. There are many such doctors, and their numbers are increasing. They are sincere and skillful, sensitive, personal and tolerant. And most importantly, they are unafraid of their own mortality. Charles Gleason was fortunate enough to have had such a doctor.

Charles had been operated on for cancer of the esophagus. Three months after his surgery, he sat in his doctor's office. He complained of intractable pain. "Dr. Noble," he said, "I don't know how much longer I have to live, but that doesn't matter right now. I want relief. Can you help me? How long I live is of no consequence right now. If I could have relief just two days a week from here on in. If I could have two hours a day of relief!"

Dr. Noble heard and understood him. "Charles," he said, "Do you want to know how long?"

Charles stammered and sputtered and then said, meekly, "Yes, Doctor, I want to know."

So Dr. Noble gently gave him what information he had. "The average life expectancy following an operation for cancer of the esophagus is one year. That doesn't mean you will only live one year. That is the average. Now, I know that you can have relief, not two days a week but seven, not two hours a day but twenty-four."

Charles Gleason was silent, pensive. "Thanks for giving it to me straight, Doctor," he said. "Now tell me, do you think I should make plans with my family to spend some time next summer at our favorite place on the lake?" It was now September.

"No, I don't think so," the doctor said. "That seems too far ahead. Do things with your family now. Make every day count. I'll help you in any way I can. Much of your stomach was

Realism About Death

removed, so you'll have to eat seven or eight small meals a day. The sphincter in your esophagus was also removed, so you must relax after a meal, or else you'll vomit. Do whatever you feel like doing...." In this way, a sensitive doctor aided a patient in charting a realistic course of action for the time left to him.

Control

Letting the patients control as much of their life as they can is to let them experience as much of life as they possibly can. Their world becomes smaller and smaller. They feel helpless in the path of an unstoppable juggernaut. And yet, given the opportunity, they can be and feel as one among the living, as validly alive as anyone else in the whole world. They need only to exerise their influence in some way, to feel that they still have some control over the events of their lives. They need to be included in decisions about their life and about the life of the family. They need to have their opinions respected.

A hospice doctor sat down with an newly arrived patient. Their simple quiet conversations went something like this:

> Patient: Do I have to eat if I don't want to?
> Doctor: No, you don't have to eat anything you don't want. But if you do want something, just ask for it.
> Patient: Do I have to take my medicine?
> Doctor: No, not if you are willing to suffer the recurring pain.
> Patient: Do I have to talk with all these visitors who come in here?
> Doctor: No. If you don't want to talk, just close your eyes and pretend you are sleeping; then no one will speak to you.

Offering constructive suggestions while permitting the patient every possible option is one way hospice caregivers help patients find meaning for their days.

Putting the House in Order

When the air is cleared of untruths and baseless hopes, a

dying patient has the opportunity to say farewell to the material world. One man contracted to have a friend keep the house, the yard and the grounds neat and trim for his wife, and to have the snow shoveled for her in the winter. Another man had his house insulated. Others try to help their wives become more conversant with insurance and retirement and other fiscal matters, although the time of terminal illness is about the most unpropitious time ever to teach a wife such things.

The need to put one's house in order, however, can run far deeper, and one must listen closely to hear those needs expressed. I met Bill in the fifth month of what would be a seventeen month terminal illness. He was interested in hospice care, and especially what "Brompton's" might do for him. It gave him a year relatively free from pain.

Bill was, in his terms, a "lapsed Catholic," and several times I asked if I could contact a priest for him. He firmly declined. He had no use for the Catholic Church, he said. After a while, the story came out. Bill had been divorced from his first wife and so had "fallen from grace." His second marriage, thirty years ago to a non-Catholic, could not be recognized by the Church. When Bill learned about his cancer, he screwed up his courage and went to the local Catholic Church to see if he could have his marriage—this happy, thirty year marriage—recognized. He told the priest that the cancer provided the motivation to try to get his marriage blessed. His first wife had been dead for many years. What, if anything, should be done?

The priest's answer, in effect, was nothing; nothing short of endless wading through ecclesiastical red tape. Bill went home in a huff, destined to be eternally miffed at this "blind and insensitive Church." Several friends suggested he ask elsewhere, that other priests were far more liberal, and that he had picked the toughest priest possible. Bill would have none of it, however. "It doesn't matter a damn!" he assured them. They all respected his integrity.

Bill entered the hospital eight months later. He roomed with a delightful Irishman by the name of Patrick Daniel O'Flaherty. Bill and Pat became close and dear friends in short order. When Pat's priest came to visit, he introduced Father O'Brien to Bill. Bill immediately mentioned that he was a former Catholic, and, with a little bidding, told the story of his frustration at the hands of the local priest. Father O'Brien said that as far as he was concerned there was no problem, and he offered to perform the wedding ceremony.

It took some time to arrange the details, but the day was finally set. Bill's wife, Mildred, looked absolutely stunning in her white dress as she stood at his bedside. By this time, he was semi-comatose. So Father O'Brien both asked and answered Bill's questions, then pronounced them husband and wife and blessed their union "in the name of the Father and of the Son and of the Holy Ghost," making the sign of the cross over him.

For the next three weeks, the last three weeks of his life, Bill was in and out of coma. But all who saw him during this time marvelled at the peace that was most obviously his. Bill had finally made things "right" with Mildred—and with something very deep within himself—thanks to a very sensitive priest.

Creativity

Far from destroying all hope and beauty for the terminally ill, an honest and supportive realism can unlock unimagined doors of creativity. A patient can communicate with another person, and with the world outside with such simple tools as crayons and paper. Those with a gift for articulation may begin using words in ways they had never dreamed possible. Creativity is an enjoyable and serendipitous discovery that enriches an otherwise sad and depressing period of one's life. When a dying person is convinced that he has something special to say to the world, and that his view of life can be enlightening to others, he might well feel freer to be creative.

Ted Rosenthal was a thirty-one year old leukemia victim. With five months to live, his penchant for noticing his surroundings and expressing his soul in song flourished. When he died, he gave his book, *How Could I Not Be Among You?*, to the world. From his vantage point, this, in part, is how life looked to Ted Rosenthal:

Kick crazily into the burrs and prickles.
Rub your back against the bark, and go ahead, peel it.
Adore the sun.
O people, you are dying! Live while you can.
What can I say?
The blackbirds blow the bush.
Get glass in your feet if you must, but take off the shoes.
Oh heed me. There is pain all over!
There is continual suffering, puking and coughing.
Don't wait on it. It is stalking you.
Tear ass up the mountainside, duck into the mist . . .
. . . Roll among the wet daisies. Blow out your lungs
Among the dead dandelion fields.
But don't delay, time is not on your side.
Soon you will be crying for the hurt, make speed.
Splash in the Ocean.
Leap in the snow.
Come on everybody! Love your neighbor
Love your mother, love your lover,
Love the man who just stands there staring.
But first, that's alright, go ahead and cry.
Cry, cry, cry your heart out.
It's love. It's your only path . . .
. . . Step lightly, we're walking home now.
The clouds take every shape.
We climb up the boulders; there is no plateau.
We cross the stream and walk up the slope.
See, the hawk is diving.
The plain stretches out ahead, then the hills, the valleys, the meadows.
Keep moving people. How could I not be among you?

Little Things

 Clearing the air of suspicions and half-truths also means making room for some delightful, sometimes raucous humor. Humorous idiosyncracies cling to a person almost to the end.
 When I first arrived at St. Christopher's I met Violet, a lady

of about fifty who was the victim of a brain malignancy. She had one of the most fetching smiles I have ever seen, and the twinkle in her eye was an immediate give away of the pixie in her. She was quick to let a person in on what she laughingly referred to as "my oddities." One of those oddities was a passion for Mars bars. She devoured them in amazing quantities and savored every slurpy mouthful. I quickly assumed coresponsibility with her husband for surreptitiously replenishing the supply of Mars bars in the top drawer of her bedside table. She would feign surprised delight at the unexplainable presence of each new cache.

I found Violet grouchy on only one occasion. I was very curious, I told her, as to why she was low that day; it was so unlike her. She told me why she was gruff, and a jolly good reason it was, too! It seems that when the nurse came in at three that morning, she had inadvertently raised the bed rail on the right side. When Violet reached out with her hand, she couldn't get beyond the bed rail. "I couldn't reach my Mars bars," she laughed, "and it kept me awake the rest of the night!"

Early in my stay at St. Christopher's I was both impressed and baffled by a quality in some of the patients that I could not identify. Slowly it dawned on me that some of them were out and out flirts. When I asked if anyone had done a study on sexuality among the dying, my English friends laughed heartily; it was so "typically American" of me to suggest a study on that subject. I never mentioned it again, not over there at least. But I kept my eyes open. I discovered back home that there are other people who feel that a healthy sexuality stays with a person almost to the end.

By sexuality I mean far more than the wrinkle of a nose or the winking of an eye. Sexuality is a state of feeling attractive, in some way, to someone else. Studies or no studies, I am confident that a healthy sexuality will flourish in an open and realistic setting, and will be suppressed, even killed, in an atmosphere where people are not honest with each other.

The need to be considered attractive is so healthy and so beautiful. Andrea, a patient at St. Christopher's was a glum and extremely tense lady. Her mother had died when she and her sister were very young. They were raised by their father who seemed never to stop reminding them that they were not attractive and that no man would ever want to marry them. And no man ever did. My telling Andrea that I thought she was a lovely person, which she was, made no impression on her. Then one day I noticed that she had just had her hair done. "Your hair looks very nice," I offered. The smile she gave in response rivaled that day's sun. When I helped her find a hairnet to wear that night, I saw an animation and a coyness in her that was present every day thereafter.

One staff member told of a man on the third floor who could scarcely move. But on one occasion when a nurse leaned over to fluff his pillow, he ran his hand up her leg. At that moment, the man's wife walked through the door and saw it all. "Good God!" she exclaimed. "He's still at it!" She brought down the house.

Free to Live . . . Free to Die

The hospice philosophy maintains that a good life deserves a good ending and a comfortable death. Death with dignity is not a defeat for the health care community; it is a tribute to the medical and caring professions. The hospice climate of openness, truth and gentleness enables patients and their families to discover untold richness in those final days. Many patients under hospice care have said that they never had it so good. Many a widow has said that providing hospice care was the best thing she could have done for her husband. Realism opens up vistas of hope, creativity and joy. Avoidance leads to the dead end of sadness and missed opportunities.

Hospice people believe that a person ought to be able to die in peace and in due season. They try to help families see that the most loving thing they can do for a patient is to let him die, not merely to perpetuate his vital signs by mechanical means. They continually pose the question, "What is best for him?" with the hope that sooner or later the family will realize that keeping him alive may be acting in *their* best interest, not his.

Any discussion about the hospice philosophy must eventually mention "The Living Will." An educational tool, its purpose is to encourage people to state, while they are in full control of their faculties and their lives, that they do not wish to have their lives artificially prolonged when there is no reasonable hope for recovery. In some states "The Living Will" is recognized as a legal document. The Society for the Right to Die foresees all other states following suit in time. But whether recognized by enactment or not, "The Living Will" provides an opportunity for a person to discuss his wishes with his family, his doctor, his minister, his lawyer and with anyone else who might someday be involved in making decisions about whether he should live or die.

What Happened to Smith?

An institution with dying patients sets the tone for acceptance or denial of death, and that tone strongly influences the behavior of its patients and their families. In most of our health care facilities, the personnel seem very blasé, very professional; they act as though they were as comfortable with death as with life.

But the denial of the reality of death runs deep in our culture, and particularly deep in our caring institutions. This denial is usually subtle enough to evade the untrained eye, but to those who see, it is glaring and stark. As one minister said about a nursing home in his community, "The denial in that place is so rampant that nobody can die openly and above board there."

Denial of death in hospitals is just as rampant. One hospital administrator described his institution's procedure when a patient dies. In a semi-private room or a ward, the nursing staff throws the curtain around the bed; they then wheel in a false-bottom cart, place the corpse in the false bottom, drape a smooth sheet over the whole thing, and then wheel it down the hall as though nothing has happened.

The assumption behind this procedure is that the other patients on the ward have no feelings about what is occurring. But these people wake up in the morning and see that "Smith" is gone. They remember that he was in bad shape last night. They wonder what happened to him, was he taken to a nursing home? They wonder if he died, and if he died they wonder if they will be treated in the same way when their time ends. "Will I become so quickly anonymous to the people who have called me by name and have taken care of me?" is the haunting question they are forced to ask themselves.

In the hospice setting, staff persons make a point of sitting down with the other patients on the ward to talk about their friend's death. They know that a death on the ward invariably sets off at least a ripple of depression. The ripple becomes a wave when the dead person was considerably younger than the survivors. The whole question of life's injustice is raised again. So staff persons share their feelings about the deceased, about how they had grown to like him, about their mixed feelings about his dying, and about life's seeming injustices. These crucial conversations are never hurried. It is important that the surviving patients have an opportunity to vent their feelings to staff persons, both about the deceased and about their depression. The ventilation process helps patients to move more quickly through their depression. They will realize once again that they will not die alone and that their bodies will be handled respectfully and lovingly.

Talk About Dying, Talk About Living

When patients and their families remove the veil of pretense and uncertainty about the patient's condition, they make it possible to talk about dying. Strangely, what dying people often ask is simply, "Am I doing it right?" They seem to want for themselves only what they can honestly and realistically expect.

The following conversation between a woman who finally accepted the fact that she would die in a few weeks and a hospice doctor is typical:

> "How long will I be around?"
> "It doesn't look as if it will be long now."
> "Am I preparing as well as can be expected?"
> "I think you are preparing extremely well."
> "Will you miss me when I die?"
> "Yes, I'll miss you; and I'll miss our friendly honest talks."

"Do you think I'll be ready when my time comes?"
"I'm certain you will be ready. I have no doubt about that. I like to think that when my time comes, I'll be as ready as you are."
"Thank you, Doctor, for helping me live."

Talk about living prevails in a hospice setting. When they have been realistic about their fate, dying patients know how to take each day as it comes better than anyone in the world. They look for ways to fill each day with as much quality as possible. It is the best of possible ways to prepare the family for what lies ahead.

5

"Family" as the Primary Unit of Caring

The wife of a dying man, who had been so poised and courageous during much of the ordeal, suddenly blurted out to a close friend, "What about me? Everybody's concerned about Harold . . . 'Is he comfortable? How are his spirits? Is there anything we can do for him?' Well, that's wonderful. But what about me? Who asks how Marjorie is doing? Who cares whether I'm tired and frustrated and at the end of my rope?" With that, she sobbed uncontrollably, the first time she had publicly lost control of her emotions during her husband's lengthy illness. The friend was wise enough and compassionate enough to assure her that she had every right to be angry, to feel alone, to be jealous of the attention given her husband, and to feel guilty about her jealousy, to cry, to be human.

The hospice movement recognizes that death is, in most instances, a social phenomenon. Consequently, the needs of the patient are viewed within the larger context of the needs of the family. For the most part, "family" means "spouse," and given the ratio of nine widows to every widower in our society, "spouse" is most often wife rather than husband. St. Christopher's prefers to identify the "Key Person," the one closest to the patient, who may or may not be the spouse. So, while other family members and friends are included in the caring, it is the "Key Person" who is of the utmost concern to hospice people, along with the patient.

There are two principle reasons for embracing the family unit of caring. First, hospice aims at enabling the family to make the patient's dying an enriching experience. The patient needs to be surrounded with love. His spouse, also, needs to know that she is not alone in her own ordeal. Together, they need to make the days count for as much *kairos* as possible. Second, hospice wants to help the family in the process of letting go of the patient. The patient will die, and the family must go on without him. So they must be supported in doing as much as they can for him while he is still alive and, at the same time, in preparing for their inevitable future.

To Build on the Positives

Every family has its own unique style. To be of greatest value and assistance, a counsellor must discover as much about that style as possible. To impose one's own style on the family, or any other style that is foreign to them, is to be of little help to the family.

One of the most helpful techniques is to get the patient and spouse to reminisce together about the enjoyable experiences of their past: how they celebrated Christmas, where they went on vacations, what the family did on weekends, and so on. The careful listener can learn much about the style of the couple's relationship: the degree of their intimacy, the extent of their willingness to share ideas and feelings, how they make decisions, how each views the other, what they laugh at and what upsets them, whether they cry together or apart or not at all. To encourage new behavior between them at this stage is totally unhelpful. They bring to this crisis the behavior that they have established through the years. And it is only out of their existing relationship that they shall discover whatever quality they will find in their last days together.

The husband of a woman with breast cancer so widespread it could not be stopped chanced to read about a local group interested in the hospice movement. He called one of the physicians mentioned in the article. Obviously distressed, he said he had a most urgent question. His wife's doctor had told him about her incurable cancer, but had warned him not to inform his wife lest she fall apart. The husband's question to the hospice physician was "Should I tell her or not?"

The physician asked the man about their relationship: were they accustomed to openness, or did they usually withhold such information from each other?

The man responded, suppressing the tears now so near the surface, "That's the problem, Doctor. We have never kept secrets from each other. Now I'm asked to be secretive in her best interest. But the deception is killing me. And it is the greatest barrier that has ever stood between us."

The physician replied, "If openness is your style, and if sharing is the accepted and expected thing between you, then by all means tell your wife." He did, much to their mutual relief.

What determines the "right thing to do?" It is certainly not the doctor's or anyone else's idea of "right," but rather the established pattern of the couple's relationship that is the final deciding factor. The life they have shared determines the "right thing to do."

Helping the patient and a "Key Person" share information with each other, to the extent they are capable of sharing, facilitates their togetherness. Information not shared contributes to separateness. Mutual emotional support, however, is even more important to family quality than is shared information. To recognize the family as the primary unit of caring is to encourage awareness of what each is enduring. The "five stages of dying" apply to the spouse or "Key Person" as surely as to the patient. The mate is also grasping at the straws of denial, hoping that there is a cure somewhere; she too may be harboring a fermenting anger, demanding to know why she, and not someone else, should be losing her husband; she too is responding emotionally in all the prescribed ways, and in a few dozen other ways nobody ever thought of. Both patient and spouse find it helpful to know that each understands the other and appreciates the enormous burden that the other must carry.

Shortly after Paul and Emily had received and shared the news of his terminal cancer, they asked me, as Hospice Chaplain, to visit them in their home. I called at the house a number of times during the following weeks. Emily was usually at work when I called, so Paul and I talked. I arranged to chat with her periodically at her place of work. Sometimes I saw them together at home.

In my conversations with Paul, I was struck by the fact that he never failed to tell me about his life insurance, about his various pensions from work, from military service and from Social Security, and of the schedule of payments to Emily after he died. A second recurring topic was Emily's testiness on weekends. "She's ok on Saturdays," he said. "But on Sundays she gets bitchier as the day wears on."

When I talked with Emily in her office she told me that Paul's preoccupation with money matters was recent and most unlike him. In fact, she said, he had always been loose with money. Now it was quite the opposite. "Money is all he talks about . . . how much he's going to leave me, how well off I'll be." She agreed with Paul's comment about her bitchiness. This was new behavior for her which she neither liked nor understood. After all, she added, she wanted their remaining days together to count for something more than discord.

The next time the three of us were together, Paul started on his favorite topic again, adding that he just couldn't get Emily to talk about this subject that was so much in her own interest. With that, Emily blustered, "For God's sake, Paul, I don't care about money. I care about you! You talk as if you were already dead!"

That statement stopped us all in our conversational tracks. No wonder she was bitchy. She wanted to have a meaningful weekend with him and he made her talk about her pending widowhood! Without fail, the weekends were painful for them both, and doubly so because they both wanted so desperately to make their remaining days together beautiful.

Lowering the Cost of Dying

One of the heaviest burdens to bear for the families of the dying in this country is the cost of hospital and medical care. The anger of dying patients and their families over excessive costs can be only partially attributed to their attempts to lash out against death. Rather, this anger rises out of a deep distrust of a health care system that prolongs life, on one hand, only to devour family assets that have taken a life's labor's to amass.

Although the hospice movement, as such, has not formally endorsed a national health program for the United States, it is important to remember that the movement began in a country where a National Health Service enables hospices to care for the dying regardless of their economic status and their ability to pay. In this country, the hospice philosophy includes reduction of the cost of dying in its concern for the family. "Brompton's Mixture" costs relatively little. The patient cost-per-day in an inpatient hospice facility falls roughly half way between the cost of treatment in a nursing home and treatment in a hospital.

However, what reduces the cost of dying most radically is home care. An active hospice program in the community can coordinate those supportive services that make it possible for a majority of terminally ill people to die at home. During the first five years of its home care program, 56% of the Connecticut Hospice's patients were able to die at home. This figure is amazingly higher than the national figures which indicate only 2% of our people dying at home.

Dying at Home

When a man dies, his widow will need to feel that she has done everything she could conceivably have done for him. This often means caring for him at home for as long as possible. There are, of course, notable exceptions, and they cry out to be honored. For one thing, the house may be too crowded. Or, the man may not want to go home to die. Perhaps he can't stand his wife, or she him, in which case sending him home would be a fate worse than that to which he is already destined. Or again, both patient and wife may acknowledge that she would simply be unable or unwilling to care for him, and that the best thing for all concerned would be to place him in the most creatively caring facility they can find.

But where physical, social and emotional conditions warrant, hospice encourages home care. The desire "to go home to die" apparently still runs deep in our culture, despite radical alterations in the pattern of American families. At home, surroundings are familiar. The family sets the daily routine and determines who visits and for how long. The wife cooks what her husband wants. At home, the family is in control.

Hospice people offer their support as it is needed throughout the dying process. They move in with their concern, and their expertise (to monitor medication, for example) and then move out, encouraging the family to do as much for themselves as they possibly can. The hospice physician makes house calls, again as needed or as promised. After all, a patient who can hardly get out of bed to go to the bathroom should not be expected to visit the doctor's office. That is a cruel and insensitive expectation.

Simple, but not Easy

The family knows they may call the hospice number at any time, day or night, around the clock and calendar. Someone will be available to listen and to offer suggestions, and, if necessary, to come to the house. Hospice people have discovered that once a family knows you are serious about being on call and available around the clock, they do not abuse the privilege. Still, the calls do come at unexpected and inconvenient hours.

One hospice worker said that the whole idea of home care is simple, but not easy. It is not easy, for example, to get out of bed at 3 a.m. to go hold the hand of a dying woman. Nor is it easy to listen to complaints that have no basis in fact but are testimony to the increasing pressure under which the spouse is living. It is a simple thing to say that the expressed complaint is a minor one. But it is sometimes difficult not to feel angry at the "impertinence."

However, the aim and task of hospice people is to help families understand their own emotional outbursts. One woman who brought her dying husband home from the hospital became extremely upset because not only would he not eat, but he also berated her as a cook. She had been having a rough time of it, feeling generally inadequate, and this outburst was almost too much for her to endure. It would seem a simple thing to tell her not to take it personally, that her husband had to direct his anger at something, and that for some reason he had chosen her cooking, but it would still be no easy matter for her. The most helpful thing the hospice visitor could say was, "You are really doing a magnificent job of caring for him under most difficult circumstances. Your husband is comfortable, clean and in his own bed. His lack of appetite is due to his illness, not your cooking."

A more difficult problem faced the hospice visitor in the home of a devoted and loving Scottish couple, both in their eighties. Since his final hospitalization, the man had lost much of his capacity for food intake. When his wife left the room, the man shook his head, wiped a tear from his eye, and said, "Aye, there's my problem. My bonnie wife. She cooks mountains of food, and when I canna eat it all, she goes off cryin'. And she dunna understand when I say it's too much fer me." No words from anyone could reach that lovely lady's confused and lonely soul.

"The Only Way"

Despite complications for the family, and despite the problems which home care creates for supporting personnel, having the patient at home is far and away the most desirable arrangement for families who are prepared to handle it.

The woman of fifty who in her lifetime had taken care of her mother, her father and her aunt during each one's terminal illness found herself and her husband free at last to fulfill some of their long-postponed dreams. But this freedom was short-lived with the discovery of a malignancy in her intestine that would soon be pronounced untreatable. Her eldest daughter's house was large, and her will to care for her mother strong. The woman lived out her final days in an upstairs room of her daughter's home. The cruel injustice of life naturally weighed heavily upon the whole family. Nonetheless, the love and devotion and caring honesty of that family gave more to visiting health care personnel than the family ever needed in return. The children in the house spent time with their grandmother each day after school and before they went to bed at night. When the woman died, her daughter thanked the hospice caregivers and said, "I'm glad we had Mom at home. We wouldn't have wanted it any other way."

Another woman who was caring for her dying husband at home said that having him in familiar surroundings with her and her two teenage sons was more than worth all the trouble: the almost total weight she supported as he shuffled to and from the bathroom, the sleepless nights, the vomiting, the incontinence of bowel and bladder, the mountains of laundry. Despite this constant toil, she felt that by being home together she and her husband were enjoying moments of intimacy that were richer than any they had ever known. "It's the only way," she smiled.

The Moral Dilemmas

Hospice workers are committed to care of the entire family unit. They, therefore, encourage each family member to "think about yourself, too." The lesson that being concerned for one's own needs is, in the end, the best thing one can do for members of the household is not readily learned. It seems, in fact, a rash contradiction. But it is invariably true, and certainly so from the patient's point of view. To know that he is not totally disrupting his family's activities removes a substantial burden from his conscience. So the wife who works must continue to work, for her own emotional health as well as to support the family during and after the crisis.

"Key Persons" faced with critical dilemmas need the ear and support of relatively objective and knowledgeable persons. One woman, for example, brought her mother home from the hospital determined to care for her until she died. Her husband and children were most agreeable and helpful. Her sister and brother, both married and living elsewhere, strongly concurred. "There is only one problem I foresee," she said. "When I can no longer feed my mother, am I legally bound to take her to a hospital or a nursing home where they can feed her through IV's?"

The hospice counsellor assured her that there were no legal requirements, but that there were emotional and moral considerations of some moment. "Are you prepared to let your mother die at home? If you don't take her to the hospital for IV's, are you prepared to face the possible censure of your husband or your children or your brother or your sister, or your aunts or uncles or cousins. . . ?"

The woman said she couldn't imagine that kind of criticism coming from her family. But after her mother had died, peacefully and at home, some of her relatives did indeed make rather cutting remarks about her "lack of concern about what happened to your dear mother." There was a rift in the family that seemed destined to last for a long time. But the woman stood her ground, convinced that she did "the right and loving thing for Mom."

Another woman confided, "I want John at home, and he wants to be at home. But I need to work. I don't think he is strong enough now to manage for himself; but he won't hear of having someone come in to stay with him while I'm gone. If he should fall and break a bone, I'd never forgive myself. What should I do?" Only she could answer the question.

Dealing with the family as the primary unit of caring means helping everyone involved in the dying process to understand the problems, to consider the possible choices, and then to support them, without qualification or reservation, in whatever choices they make.

Religious Ritual

Because it is affiliated with the Church of England, St. Christopher's Hospice stresses the importance of religion in life. Chapel services are held each day for the staff. Sunday services attract patients of all faiths. Some of them walk to the chapel; some come in wheelchairs; some have their beds rolled in. Personal religious needs and preference can also be met because of the willing flexibility of the hospice program. On one occasion at St. Christopher's, a Pentecostal family asked their minister to say prayers of healing over their loved one. On another day, a group of some ten to twelve gypsies gathered prayerfully around the bed of one of their number.

"Lady"

From time to time, the term "Key Person" needs a broad interpretation. One forty-two year old woman at St. Christopher's had been abandoned by her husband some twelve years earlier. He had moved to another city, lived with another woman and fathered two sons by her. When the second woman died, the man brought his two young sons "home," only to find his wife in the last stages of cancer and living in indescribable filth and squalor. He contacted the Public Health authorities who arranged for the woman to be admitted to St. Christopher's.

The woman, wasted and gaunt, showed no emotion in her new, bright, clean, friendly surroundings. She spoke blandly of her life; she demonstrated no feeling of any kind toward the man who had deserted her and the two boys who were not her own. No one could coax the faintest smile from her. Finally, a social worker stumbled upon a successful plan. The woman had a dog that had shared her misery with her, an ugly terrier-sort of mongrel named "Lady." The staff arranged a visit to the Hospice by "Lady," and that first visit was repeated every night while the woman remained alive. A friend drove into the Hospice parking lot and opened the car door. "Lady" raced to the entrance and danced madly in the doorway until someone let her in. She then dashed across the lobby, down the hall, up the stairs to the second floor, down the hall to the third ward, into the ward, across the floor to her mistress's bed. She leaped up on the bed and licked the woman's face while an ecstatic tail wagged deliriously. The woman took "Lady" in her arms. And for the first and only time that day, and each day after, she smiled!

Life for the Living

In time, the patient dies; but hospice care for the family continues. Everything is now geared toward helping the family work through their period of grief. Life can never be the same for them, but with some help they can, in time, discover a way to live meaningfully in the world.

Bereavement experts reassure us that shock and numbness

and pining are normal for the grieving person. They also declare that our society does not know how to help the widowed. Death is both awkward and taboo in our death-denying culture. Consequently, the bereaved must, for the most part, go it alone on the painful course.

Janet's husband died of Hodgkin's Disease. Three months after his death, she suffered severe back pains. The pains were located in the same area of the back where her husband's pain had been centered. A doctor's examination turned up no physiological cause of the pain. Janet discovered lumps on her body, identical to those that were first symptomatic of her husband's fatal illness. Thorough examinations produced nothing. Both Janet and her doctor agreed that hers were sympathetic symptoms. She knew it was true. She was glad it was true. But as the lumps and backaches persisted, she realized that she was having a most difficult time of letting go of her dead husband.

Many widowed persons have mistakenly withdrawn or have driven people away by their abrasiveness in order to avoid sharing experiences with people who, they are sure, won't understand them. When the friend of one widow insisted she tell her story, the woman told of her hearing her husband speak to her, and even of feeling his body next to hers in bed. She complained about not being able to get up in the morning and of an inability to make decisions. She was baffled by it all, she said, and feared she was losing her mind. It was a wise and caring friend who replied, "It's called grief, and it's as normal as breathing."

Bereavement is a painful and lonely process. However, most people do come out at the other end of the long tunnel, though each person's style and timing will be unique, with a little help from people who understand and care.

The Grieving Family and the Hospice Staff

When a young woman died at St. Christopher's, the medical staff immediately assured the family that everything possible had been done for her right up to the end. The family—her husband, father, and mother—knew it was true. They were then asked to come back the next morning to pick up the woman's things.

When they arrived the next day, they were taken to a quiet room where they were greeted by one of the doctors, the head nurse and the chaplain. Once again, the doctor said that the hospice staff had done everything they could, and then added a word of praise for the obvious love and devotion the family had for each other. They had certainly been faithful in their visiting.

Tea was served. The head nurse then gave the family the woman's effects. It might have been a holy ritual. She handled each item with reverence and respect and gave it to the appropriate person: the ring to the husband, the housecoat to the mother, and so on. When the ritual ended, the local funeral director came in and, in the presence of the hospice personnel, who gave the impression they had nothing more to do that morning, helped the family make the funeral arrangements.

As the family walked outside to their car after their month-long experience at St. Christopher's, the father, a stoical man of few words, said to the chaplain, "You know, I dislike hospitals. I have often thought that I would never want to be a patient in one of them. But if I could come to a place like this. . . ."

Team Initiative

"Please call me if I can be of help" may be a sincere offer extended to a widowed person, but it rarely gains a response. The widowed, by and large, do not ask people to help them. One woman, whose husband Jake had been dead for three months, said that none of her friends ever mentioned him any more. "So I don't mention him either. After all, I need my friends, and they don't want to be around a person who is always talking about the dead." But it was clear that she wanted more than anything to talk with someone about Jake.

Hospice people remind the family that they may call at any time. In fact, they are encouraged to keep in touch. But hospice people also realize that they must be persistent, and they take the initiative in a number of ways. For example, if at all possible, someone from hospice attends the funeral. Those workers closest to the family during the illness may send a note or card to the spouse on such special occasions as holidays, birthdays, or the anniversary of the patient's death.

Dr. Colin Murray Parkes, staff psychiatrist at St. Christopher's, has devised a simple system for anticipating how families will cope with loss. Shortly after the patient dies, the head nurse checks a number of items on a card questionnaire. Categories include such items as the number of children at home, the occupation, if any, of the "Key Person," the degree of clinging or pining or anger or self-reproach displayed during the terminal illness, the relationship of the family members after the patient's death. Each item is given a value and a tally is made. If the total of the values is high, it is conceded that the family may need to be followed up with more than average support. A low score indicates the family will probably cope well without much outside aid.

Staff persons meet at least once each month to discuss contacts they have had with families of former patients to ascertain if anything further can be done to help them.

St. Christopher's also offers "The Pilgrim Club," a monthly nighttime social affair in the family room of the Hospice. "Key Persons" of patients are invited to attend. "The Pilgrim Club" gatherings are command performances for all staff people: administrators, doctors, nurses, porters, social workers, chaplains, orderlies. In short, everyone is expected to make an earnest effort to attend. For this is a kind of homecoming night for people whose only pleasant memories of the past few years are of relationships formed and maintained at the Hospice.

Bereavement support, like support of the patient and the family, is a team effort in the hospice program. That team approach, however, is not easily achieved. It requires an appreciation of each person's contribution, a willingness to learn together and a structure of continuing mutual support.

6

Staff Support

The hospice movement defies the contemporary myth that to be professional one cannot be compassionate, a myth that has blossomed with the increase of sophisticated medical technology.

At one time, medical students were chosen partly because they were sensitive and person-oriented. Now, they are chosen exclusively because of their intelligence, on the basis of their potential as technicians. Before medical technology boomed, doctors had themselves to give, frequently at the patient's bedside. Today the doctor offers, for the most part, only his considerable skills. He is a modern medical Delphic Oracle, the unquestioned Last Word who is best served by blind obedience.

Doctor and patient were once friends, colleagues, teammates who were mutually concerned about the patient and his family as persons. Today, the patient's *illness*, not the patient, is the object of the medical team's technical diagnosis, treatment and experimentation. The suggestion that someone else down the line will benefit from the doctor's experiments on him is scant comfort to the patient as a human being who is faced with death.

Whatever Happened to Compassion?

A young doctor, recently exposed to the hospice philosophy of care for the dying, admitted to a radical change of viewpoint.

"Before hospice," he said, "I would have been ashamed to admit compassion for a patient. We doctors are educated in skills, treatment, curing. The role models we saw as students were unfeeling, almost calloused. I thought that to be compassionate was to be unprofessional."

To fly in the face of the myth is risky business, for compassion is broadly unacceptable in most professional ranks. A hospice social worker, who strongly identified with the anger and the frustration of a cancer patient she was visiting regularly, expressed to another social worker her own anger at being unable to help the patient. The colleague's response was typically and frighteningly professional: "You seem to get involved with your clients. Do you think you're in the wrong work?"

Who can afford to risk being considered unprofessional by one's peers? A consulting psychiatrist working with a group of nurses in a hospital told of a conversation with one nurse who confessed to being deeply grieved by the death of a child. "She began sobbing softly," he said. "The longer she talked, the harder she cried. I tried to reassure her, but it was largely in vain. She didn't need my words. I wanted to hold her, as I would my daughter, but I couldn't." Then he reasoned, pleadingly, "Why can't we do for each other, as caregivers, what we would do for the dying patient?"

Hospice care aims at restoring compassion in the health care community as a professionally valid ingredient, as acceptable and necessary as any skill, technique or intelligence. This is not to suggest that hospice care is mostly sentimentality. Quite the contrary, hospice emphasizes the importance of coordinating the skills and insights of all applicable disciplines on behalf of the patient and his family. For example, the zealous development of a method of controlling chronic pain is sophisticated pharmacology, not mere well-wishing. Again, the determination of family strengths and weaknesses requires an intelligent and skillful sociology, not simply warm feelings. But along with the requirement of intelligence in meeting human needs, hospice would reinstate compassion and deep concern for the whole person as a professionally legitimate practice. It is this combination of head and heart that one senses immediately at St. Christopher's and other hospice organizations. Of that combination, George F. Will wrote in the January 9, 1978 issue of *Newsweek*, "St. Christopher's staff generally has the placidness of a gentle river which, over time, cuts canyons in granite."

It is not by sheer accident that a hospice staff combines compassion, skill and devotion into a finely tuned instrument. Nor is it a simple matter to create the kind of supportive climate in which a person may share deep stresses with colleagues and not be denigrated as a professional. The strategy begins with the selection of personnel.

The Selection Process

If intelligence and skill were clearly paramount in determining who is best qualified for hospice caring, the selection process would be relatively easy. First, academic degrees, experience, publications and scholarship rankings would be considered. Then, the applicants with highest composite scores would be selected.

Of course, no hiring is that simple, and it becomes especially complicated when such intangible qualities as dedication, emotional stability, compassion, and ability to work with others must be gauged. But hospice staffs must be long on the intangibles as well as on the skills, and it is the intangibles that require a good deal of intuition on the part of the administrator.

It would seem probable that the person who had cancer would be the person most helpful to another cancer patient. I have a good friend in that category, a doctor who is active in the hospice movement. But I know another doctor, a cancer surgeon, whose own brother has waged a successful battle against cancer, but who is still so frightened of the disease that he can only encourage his patients to deny reality. These two medical professionals possess comparable skill (the latter actually supersedes the former because of his technological specialization) and are veterans of similar crises, yet they are complete opposites in other crucial matters. The former relates warmly to patients. The latter is preoccupied with surgical processes and the treatment of diseases.

Thus, simply because doctors or nurses may be cancer specialists does not automatically qualify them for hospice care of terminally ill patients. Specialists have been trained to fight illness, to cure and to rehabilitate the patient. They may be wanting rather desperately in compassion for the patient as a living human being.

Dedication to human needs ranks high on the list of criteria for hospice service. Dr. Tom West, Deputy Director at St. Christopher's, was once a medical missionary in Africa. His religious devotion and his unquestioned professional skill combine to make him an ideal hospice doctor. By the same token, a hospice nurse of zealous religious bent makes "conversion" of the patient a major aim of her care. She is unsatisfied in her work and looks toward a foreign mission task for her church. She is undeniably an excellent nurse, but religion, for her, is more important than nursing. She very frankly and admittedly has a hard time seeing people die "without the Lord."

Sympathy for others, arising out of critical personal loss, can be a valuable asset for hospice service. Leaders of community widow-to-widow programs realize that no one can help a widow like another widow who has successfully worked through her grieving. They will not involve a widow as counsel and support for another widow unless she has been widowed for at least two years. However, a hospice program is no substitute for creative bereavement; it is always possible that a well-meaning and sympathetic caregiver may try to atone for unresolved guilt by over-protecting and controlling a patient like a mother hen.

Unresolved guilt is difficult to identify in an interview with a prospective caregiver. It is even more difficult to identify such guilt in compassionate acts. But its symptoms are frequently manifested in a "knowing what's best for him" attitude. For example, the advice to a recently widowed woman to "sell your house and make a new start for yourself" may reflect more the counsellor's unresolved guilt over having neglected a terminally ill loved one than a wisely determined formula for the widow.

Too Much Love

A hospice staff person's emotional wholeness and inner security help patients and families exercise maximum control over their situation. These qualities also greatly reduce the staff person's need to be personally gratified from participation in a hospice program.

Next to being free from pain, nothing is so crucial to the quality of patients' days as control over their own activities. If hospice programs can be faulted at all, it is at the point of being so loving, kind and thoughtful that the patient and his family are deprived of the right of complaint. It is not unusual for hospice patients to say, "These people are so kind. How could I possibly gripe?" Indeed, complaining would seem to be the height of ingratitude. On the other hand, a stifled complaint might be the result of a "love-'em-to-death" attitude by caregivers. Too much kindness can destroy the patient's right to express his anger as he stands in the path of certain death.

The food at St. Christopher's is excellent. When rating it as institutional food, one must speak in superlatives. Every effort is made to serve the patients their meals swiftly, efficiently, considerately and with regard for personal tastes and palates. That effort is generally appreciated by the patients. One evening, however, the staff in one of the ward kitchens was astonished when a male patient came careening in, waving his plate of food precariously. He shouted, "What kind of food is this, anyway? I'll tell you what it is. It's shit-food." With that, he flung his plate into the sink and stalked out of the room. The staff doubled over with laughter! They recognized his need to exercise some control over the situation, even if his criticisms were ill placed. They might have taken the slap as a personal criticism or as a rejection of their diligent devotion, but they knew better. They were also personally strong enough to laud his defiance.

Personal ego strength, the quality of "having it all together," is a major criterion by which hospice staff are selected. "Having it all together" implies having come to grips with one's own mortality. One hospice chaplain-in-training frequently expressed displeasure at his inability to get a patient he was seeing to talk about the afterlife. "I don't know what he is thinking," he lamented. "There must be many things going through his mind. I know there would be a lot of questions *I* would be asking if *I* were in his bed. But he never says anything about what he expects after he dies...." In time, the budding counsellor realized that there might be a very simple explanation for that patient's not talking about immortality, namely, that it was not a relevant topic to him. Why, then, the counsellor's concern about the patient's silence? The answer came out in a team conference one day: "I guess I'm worried for myself."

"Miss Jane"

The caregiver's biases, especially the well-intentioned ones, are often a stumbling block to creative care. The staff person's preoccupations can prompt unnecessary and inappropriate actions which a patient may neither want nor need. The religiously oriented, for example, discover a multitude of cases in point in their specialized field of interest, and their biases can be as disconcerting to the patient as a doctor's denial of death or a nurse's anger over a patient's complaint.

One of the first requests I received as Visiting Chaplain at St. Christopher's came from several staff persons. They asked me to visit a woman who was not on my ward because, they said, she was "Noncomformist," the sectarian label which is applied to Protestants other than members of the Church of England. "Miss Jane" was in her mid-90s, almost totally blind and just as deaf. Needless to say, I needed some help in communicating with her. The idea was that "Miss Jane" might have some special thing to say to me, since our religious viewpoints were supposedly somewhat similiar.

"Miss Jane" was a delightful lady. She had a delicious sense of humor. She also lived up to the staff's advanced billing as a truly devout soul. We had our most moving moments together saying The Lord's Prayer and when I read, and she recited, the Twenty-third Psalm. I was very glad they had asked me to see her. She *was* a special person.

But my satisfaction was countered by a subtle and prodding

interrogation by the people who had introduced us. In our staff conversations, the question of whether she had asked to receive Holy Communion surfaced repeatedly. I said that the subject had never come up in our conversations. They responded with a sense of urgency; they felt "Miss Jane" both wanted and needed the sacrament. I agreed, therefore, to be specific and direct in my next visit with her.

"Do you want to take Communion?" I asked bluntly, as we "Nonconformists" are wont to do.

"Good heavens!" she laughed. "Have they got to you, too?"

Then she added laboriously, but never without a twinkle in her deep blue eyes, "They've been after me to receive the sacrament ever since I came in here. I don't need it. My communion is with God. I love him. I trust him. I'm ready to go to him. And I know he's about ready to receive me. So why do I need the sacrament?"

"You don't, of course," I said, with great relief.

"But I'll do it if they insist. Maybe I should, to make them happy. They have been very good to me."

In the coffee room that afternoon, someone asked me if I had broached the subject with "Miss Jane."

"Yes," I replied. "She doesn't want it, and I can't give it to her if she doesn't want it. She says she is communing with God already, and that seems to be sufficient for her."

The matter was dropped, but not to the complete satisfaction of those who had brought their sacramental bias to "Miss Jane's" bedside.

Although it is a church-oriented institution, St. Christopher's deliberately sets a low religious profile. The avowed stance there is to let the patient and the family determine the role formal religion is to play in their last days together. Nevertheless, the biases sometimes are stronger than the avowals. That is normal. But the biases must be looked for in the staff selection process.

My own biases looked me squarely in the eye early in my stay at St. Christopher's, thanks to the staff psychiatrist Colin Murray Parkes. Dr. Parkes conducted a weekly patients' group which was attended by both in- and out-patients. The members of the group talked about anything they wished. One week, for instance, the mother of a twenty-two year old woman who had died at St. Christopher's was the featured speaker. Since her daughter's death, the woman had been writing poetry. She read her poems publicly for the first time that day; she has since published her first book of poems. Another day, several patients brought in some things they had written since their illnesses. And one day I, an American minister, was the speaker.

Dr. Parkes had asked me to tell the group why I had come to St. Christopher's. It was a tough assignment for me. I found myself wanting to protect them, or so I thought. I used general terms and evasive language throughout my speech. I had come, I said, "to meet people in the world-renowned institution . . . to learn about the program . . . to meet the patients . . . and to learn from them so I might be a more effective minister back home."

After the meeting, Dr. Parkes asked me why I hadn't told them why I had really come to St. Christopher's. When I replied with my "to protect them" stance, he gently and forthrightly stated that the patients could take realism. "If you had told them you were here to learn something about what it is like to be dying and to learn how to make these last few days count for something and how people can die with dignity, they would have understood perfectly," he said. "They wouldn't have been upset in the least."

Colin Murray Parkes is a man who makes a decisive point without being painfully incisive. I got his message: it was *my* problem.

Diminishing World, Few People

Compassion, skill and inner stability top the list of criteria for hospice caregivers. After these, one need remains: a person must be able to work well with others, and to do so in an extraordinary sense. In an atmosphere in which dedicated caregivers strive earnestly, at times burn, to be helpful, it is crucial that they be able to accept their limitations. It is no reflection upon the caregiver's usefulness to be unable to meet every last need of the patient and his family. One wants and, to

Staff Support

a point, needs to feel that one has enough to offer and give in any situation. But the patient is the one who finally decides who is most helpful and who is not. And the patient's decision is the final authority.

As the patient's world diminishes, the number of people around him decreases. Many friends and relatives excused themselves earlier along the road of his illness. Now, near the end of that road, he has strength to invest in only a few relationships. He alone chooses those relationships. Consequently, the caregiver needs to learn quickly to accept the fact that someone else may be chosen by the patient as the one to whom he will remain closest.

No Hierarchy on the Ward

Hospice dedicates the resources of a variety of disciplines and skills to the patient and the family. The program is completely a team effort. The team motif has sounded since the first day of inpatient care at St. Christopher's: "There is no hierarchy on the ward!" The hospice tries to impress that fact continuously upon both staff and patients. In America, the quickly identifiable symbol of nursing rank is the cap. In British hospitals it is the belt. At St. Christopher's that symbol is removed in order to remind the staff of the equal regard their unique services and opinions will receive, and to suggest to patients that a cooperative and coordinated program supports them.

In those first days of activity at St. Christopher's, when the ideal of hospice care shone most brilliantly, the motif was readily and easily embodied. The staff was small, communication was almost constant, and mutual respect among professional friends flowed naturally. Since that time, the team has expanded to two hundred people. What, then, has happened to the concept of "no hierarchy"? Amazingly, it remains essentially intact. To be sure, a patient quickly separates the doctors from the nurses, the volunteers from the orderlies, a chaplain from a pharmacologist or a porter. And there can be no question of authority or hierarchy when Dr. Saunders is on the ward, or in the dining room. She has earned a respect which, at times, she finds a bit awkward. At the same time, however, top staff members, Dr. Saunders included, do ask for opinions about patients and families. And they do listen carefully, especially when a patient's condition is the topic. There is a broad respect for each person's observations and opinions.

Staff Notes

St. Christopher's staff use a special sheet on which they note conversations they feel could prove relevant for the care of the patient. An example of the process is this composite list of conversations, each with a different member of the staff, the last of which took place with a doctor:

> Alice Bloom, age 63, was admitted on June 1, 1974 with cancer of the intestine; her admission form stated she had been told nothing about her illness prior to her coming to the hospice.
> June 1. "Are we incurables here?" When asked why she had asked that question, she replied, "I was just thinking."
> June 14. The patient told me she wasn't feeling well today, then added forcefully, "I'm not worried about it because I know I'm getting better."
> June 17. "Do you know what is wrong with me? Yesterday I thought I was dying. I suppose nobody really knows what's wrong with me, do they?"
> June 17. "I thought this was a convalescent home . . . I wish they would tell me if I've got cancer . . . people do get better from that, don't they?"
> June 17. The patient was gently told she has cancer and is dying.
> "Will you keep me here?"
> "Yes, of course."
> "Do I have to eat?"
> "No."
> "Good. Can I sleep?"
> "As much as you like."
> "Oh good!"
> The patient told her family today. She seems relieved and unafraid to die.

Input by Local Clergy

If the patient is affiliated with a church or temple, his spiritual advisor should be invited to be a part of the caring team. His perspective can be invaluable, for he has seen and known the patient and the family for a long time, and he will be the family's friend years after their hospice experience. He probably married the patient and his wife. He laughed with them and held their babies. He prayed with them when their children were ill. He held his breath with them when their teenagers were asserting their independence. He officiated at the children's weddings. He knows where the family has been and what has transpired before this crisis. He can, therefore, enlighten the hospice team on the strengths of the patient and on the positive ingredients in the family relationships.

Of course, many ministers, priests and rabbis will not want to be an active team member, but they will nevertheless appreciate the invitation. They will also undoubtedly appreciate the fact that a hospice chaplain, a specialist, who can act for them in these special circumstances, is always available.

Cottage by the Sea

The team approach in hospice care dedicates everything to the patient and the family, and little or nothing to the caregiver as a person. Any staff person looking for special consideration which interferes in any way with the ongoing program will be refused. "Neither the hospice nor the patient owes you a thing," is the stark, thoroughly professional theme.

On the other hand, the hospice organization must be sensitive to the emotional needs of its dedicated staff. Hospice staff persons require more frequent vacations. Administrators of the program, therefore, encourage a variety of vacation possibilities for their staff. For example, a grateful family has offered their seaside cottage as a vacation retreat to St. Christopher's personnel. It is free of charge and is available to anyone of the staff; a reasonable advance reservation is the only requirement.

Training the Staff

An orientation program for hospice caregivers includes an elevation of each person's strengths and an acceptance of each person's limitations. Team-building requires the full participation of every team member, including the hospice doctors.

In a hospital setting, there is no democracy. The buck of decision stops with the doctor. He has the final say. In the hospice program, however, the doctor is only one member of a professional team, one voice contributing to a group decision. That fact can be both a relief and an affront to a doctor. If he is reluctant to surrender "the last word," he detracts from the hospice team concept of caring. But by relinquishing some of his authority, he no longer carries the sole responsibility for weighty decisions. He does not have to play God.

Mrs. Smythe was a patient whose pain had inexplicably worsened. The Medical Director and the nursing staff of the hospice program discussed such alternative ways of keeping her comfortable as increased "Brompton's" dosage strength, palliative radiation treatments and the severing of a nerve. The doctor had a preference among the possible medical procedures, but the nurses' data on Mrs. Smythe's attitude and general morale were equally important. Together, the team made a joint decision which was recommended to both the patient and the family.

Another patient, Mrs. Keening, had contracted pneumonia. The question before the team was: "Do we put her on antibiotics, or do we keep her comfortable and let her die?" There are no automatic answers to such questions in the hospice philosophy. Sometimes, the best medical procedure is to let the patient die; sometimes it is not. The social worker was asked about the family's readiness to let Mrs. Keening die. The chaplain said Mrs. Keening seemed to be at peace with herself and had accepted her death. Rarely does a hospice staff put the burden of this kind of decision on the family. The staff wrestles with the alternatives and comes to a consensus. Then, and only then, will they discuss the problem and the recommended course of action, or inaction, with the family. It is rare instance when a family refuses that kind of counsel, or fails to appreciate the courage of a sensitive staff that is willing to shoulder the onus of so serious a decision.

Vaccinated Vultures

Orientation and training of the entire team is also essential in order to prevent well-intentioned but ill-informed caregivers from contributing to the problems of the patient and family instead of to their solution.

In recent years, since the doors to the foreboding mausoleum in which the subject of death and dying was entombed have been thrown open, there has been a headlong rush into the field. Colleges, hospitals, mental health centers and churches offer courses in death and dying. Libraries and book stores have opened whole new sections for death and dying tomes. The general effect of bringing the subject to light has been indisputably salutary. However, two serious problems have also emerged.

For one thing, many teachers and authors on the subject have neither submitted themselves to the discipline of team questioning nor logged any appreciable personal time with dying patients and their families. They have read the literature and attended the workshops and written term papers, but rarely have they sat with a patient in helpless silence. It is lamentable that many people who just walk through a hospice facility on a quick tour assume an air of expertise on hospice care.

A second problem arising from the spate of interest in death and dying is a mass of "knowledgeable" caregivers who are rushing in to have dying patients tell them what it is like to be dying. Having been vaccinated by reading about the dying process, contraction of the disease called "Learning" becomes extremely difficult. One person has expressed concern over this "horde of death and dying vultures who can't wait to get into the sickroom to hover over the deathbed and analyze the patient's progress throughout the five stages of dying." That appraisal may be too harsh, but there is no doubt that there is a wave of only slightly exposed "experts" who feel they have more to offer than to gain at the bedside of the dying person.

Existential Anxiety

No caregiver can honestly say to a dying patient, "I understand your denial." The caregiver's "understanding" is theoretical; the patient's understanding is existential and real. This difference in perspective indicates a central problem in care giving. There is an unbridgeable chasm between the dying man's reality and the healthy man's theory.

Consequently, it is not by a recitation of "the five stages of dying," or of any other observed phenomena, that one human being makes genuine contact with another human being. Genuine contact can only be made at the existential level, at the level of human existence and experience.

Everyone, living or dying, can ask the question, "What does it mean to exist, to be?" Unless caregivers have asked that question about their own lives, they cannot begin to appreciate that every day the patient is asking, "What does my life mean?" More specifically, the patient asks, "Is this what dying is all about?"

So the hospice team orientation surely ought to begin, not with a catechismal recitation of "the five stages of dying," nor with any evaluation of patient behavior, but with each person's humanness. For the greatest gift anyone can give to any other person is the gift of self. Presence. Listening. Identification. Caregivers may not be dying, but they are human. Patients are dying, but they are also human.

What, then, does it mean to be human, both to the patient and to the caregiver? The late philosopher-theologian Paul Tillich suggests that to be human is to be anxious. This concept is an excellent starting definition. Tillich spoke of existential anxiety. Because we exist, we are anxious about three things. We are anxious, first, about the meaning of our lives. Viktor Frankl, writing out of his experience in a concentration camp, is convinced that having something to live for—meaning, purpose—is our greatest single motivation for life. Without meaning, we have nothing to live for.

"What is the meaning of life?" is one of the perennial human questions. At every stage of our lives, indeed, every day of our lives, we ask the question. What does it mean to be a three-year-old? What does it mean to be a teenager? To be married? To be fifty? Retired? A grandparent? What does it mean to be dying? Unfortunately, there is no one correct and final answer to this question for the individual person or for the human race. That is why we are anxious about the meaning of life. And that, says Tillich, is why it is human to be anxious.

Those dying patients on Ward 4 are all asking, "What does my life mean today?" We can only sense their struggle when we ask the same serious question for ourselves: "What does it mean to be alive today?"

Tillich suggests the anxiety over guilt as a second anxiety. Everyone's life is loaded with "ifs." From early on, we have been making decisions. But every yes creates a no. Who knows how our lives might have been different if the noes had been yesses, or if some of the yesses had been noes! And what of other yesses, and other noes? We can never know. Every parent understands that. We can read all the books on child-rearing, and follow the best advice with the best intentions and still wonder if we are doing the right things for and to our children.

St. Paul put his finger on the problem of guilt in *Romans* 7:19. Somewhat loosely translated, Paul says, "The good I want to do I never seem to do; and what I don't want to do is what I always seem to end up doing."

The problem of guilt is expressed in every decision families have to make for the well-being of a patient. Never knowing what is absolutely the best thing to do, partly because their own best interests are involved, they are always confronted with the question of what might have been if other choices had been made. Anxiety over guilt is also a major block in the bereavement process for survivors who try to do for the deceased what they did not or could not do for him while he was still alive.

The third existential anxiety centers on death. Since none of us has been on the other side of the grave, death confronts us as a total mystery. Voices from beyond may allay the fears of some. Theological formulas about immortality will help others. But there are no certainties beyond the grave. Death remains far more a question mark than an exclamation.

We know this life, this world. And it is a threatening experience, to say the least, to lose what we know and to face what we do not know. According to such existential philosophers as Albert Camus, death is what makes life absurd. In one bold stroke, death wipes out a life, a total life. Death steals from the world the accumulated intelligence, wisdom, leadership, companionship and appreciation of life that *is* a human being. Absurd! No wonder, then, that because we are human we are anxious about death—and about the dying process, since that, too, is a new experience.

The patient with a week to live and the family standing at his bedside have at least this much in common with each other, and with the caregiver as well: they are all human beings, and they are all anxious about life's meaning, about guilt and about death. So the subject of one's humanness is the place to begin in the orientation of a hospice staff. For humanness is what all caregivers have in common, with each other and with those who need their caring.

The Staff Support System

A small community hospital presented a panel on team caring to a group of interested citizens. The four panelists—doctor, nurse, chaplain, social worker—spoke of the patient's multiple needs and of ways they, as a team, combined to try to meet those needs. During the audience question period, someone asked where the team members went to have their personal emotional and psychological needs met. "How do you handle the enormous inner pressures you must all feel from time to time?" the questioner asked.

The nurse said she had an understanding husband who encouraged her to vent her feelings at home. The social worker and chaplain met regularly with professional colleagues. The doctor replied, "There is no place to go." Elaborating, he added that, of course, he found support from fellow physicians occasionally and incidentally. However, his initial response was one of isolation.

Crying in All the Wrong Places

The professional caregivers' need for a reliable support system in which to air their feelings and personal concerns was demonstrated by a young nurse who confessed, "I seem to be crying in all the wrong places." Working with the terminally ill, she would frequently cry with the patients and with their families. The problem created by her tears was that the patient and family felt they needed to support her.

Under less stressful circumstances, their support of the nurse might be considered quite therapeutic for them. But when a life is about to end, the family's entire strength is focused on themselves. They have no energy, at that point, for care *giving*.

A hasty appraisal might judge the nurse to be in the wrong profession, even though she was an excellent nurse—skillful, compassionate and intelligent, a hard worker and a good team person. Or, she might be thought to be under too much pressure working with the terminally ill.

Both diagnoses could be accurate. But both suggestions might also prematurely result in the unfortunate loss of a considerable talent on the ward. A third opinion might harness the nurse's compassion for her patients and enable her to realize her full potential as a topnotch caregiver to the terminally ill. A professional support system that would allow her to express her feelings about her patients to her peers without loss of professional esteem could well be the best solution to her problem.

Crying with patients and their families is not, in itself, unprofessional. It may even be totally and beautifully uplifting. Early in my stay at St. Christopher's, I was asked to read prayers of commendation for the dead and of support for the living at the bedside of a young woman who had just died. As I walked into the ward, I saw the woman's family standing around her, and one of the hospice doctors sitting on the bed, holding the dead woman's hand, and crying. His tears in concert with those of the family, expressed both sadness and relief. They seemed thoroughly appropriate, not tears that invited or required the sympathy and support of the family.

An effective support system frees caregivers to offer more of themselves to their patients. Far from reinforcing the myth that it is unprofessional to cry, a support system provides a nonjudgmental climate in which professional peers can be completely honest with each other about their feelings of helplessness, anger, frustration and humility. Such a system serves as an emotional release that sends caregivers back into the ward with all their compassion and skills intact and with their emotions harnessed for appropriate expression. The support system makes it possible for them to cry in all the right places.

"Unfinished Business"

Support groups do not just happen. They require a regular meeting schedule and faithful attendance by participants. The support process is aimed at creating, building and maintaining trust among staff members, to establishing a climate of openness and mutual acceptance in which no subject is taboo. The process can be facilitated by having an observer aboard who is conversant in the dynamics of human relationships. That, however, is only a requirement for accelerating the process. Regular meeting times and faithful attendance are the more essential requirements. To obtain the maximum benefit, groups should be kept small—six to twelve participants.

St. Christopher's provides working time off for four weekly group meetings. Participants need only to determine if ward schedules permit an hour's absence by one or two staff members. In other hospice programs, leadership is provided for groups which meet after working hours; while in still others, lunch periods are extended by mutual agreement. In any event, sessions need to last at least an hour. It frequently takes that long for the dynamics to stir and for the group to process its experiences in order to learn from them.

The supportive process and the individuals in the group are best served by beginning each session with "unfinished business": What issues from the last meeting have the members been thinking about during the week? or what has happened on the wards that has raised some questions which group members would like to discuss? Frequently, there is a ready response, and sometimes it leads the group into unexplored territory.

In one group, a nurse responded to the invitation for "unfinished business" with, "Just the other day, Mr. Evans said he wanted to end it all. I tried to kid him out of it, but I quickly realized he was serious. I didn't know what to do. I was scared, so I got out of there in a hurry. After that, every time I had to go into his room, I dreaded it. He must have noticed my discomfort because he didn't look at me or speak to me. This is not good. I'm not helping him one bit. Did anybody else ever have a patient talk about suicide? How did you handle it?"

After a moment or two of awkward silence, others in the group admitted to having similar reactions when patients broached the subject of suicide. They talked for a while about depression in the terminally ill. They agreed that, in the future, the situation called for a sympathetic ear and some quality time sitting on the edge of the patient's bed, just listening, without judgment or advice.

When the subject had been helpfully if not thoroughly processed, the leader asked, "Has anybody here ever contemplated suicide?" With that, the nurse who had introduced the subject began sobbing. "Yes!" she cried. "When my husband left me I wanted desperately to kill myself. The only thing that saved me was my little boy. What would he do without me?"

Silence. Interminable silence.

Then she added, "Oh, I'm so glad I didn't do it. But I was all alone in the world. Except my son!" Then, "You know, I've never told anyone before. I've felt so guilty, so dirty."

The person on either side of her each took a hand in their own.

"How do you feel now?" asked the leader.

"Oh, so much better!" she said, beaming.

"Do you suppose your pent-up guilt had anything to do with your avoiding Mr. Evans?"

"There's no doubt in my mind about that," she said. Then she looked about the room, smiling at each of her friends. "I'm really looking forward to going to see him this afternoon."

Her group had made it possible for her to cry in the right place by dealing with her "unfinished business."

In another group, someone quoted from an article in which a nurse had said, "I just hope he doesn't die on my shift." There was a healthy guffawing from these people who recognized those words from their own past. One nurse, however, did not laugh.

"I still feel that way," she said, somewhat embarrassed. "But it's not because of what you think. You see I'm afraid if patients die on my shift I'll have to stay over and do the paper work on them... and I really can't do that." She then told them about an extremely difficult marriage situation that required all her non-working time and energy.

She left the meeting that day with the offer from her colleagues to fill in for her whenever she needed to leave. More than that, she left with newly-found support in her own personal trials.

More than Ships in the Night

Fruits of the support system are also manifested outside the group setting. Hospice people are more than "ships that pass in the night" to each other when they meet outside the hospice walls. In Victoria Station I saw one of the women who worked in the kitchen of our ward at the hospice. She walked up to me with her husband and, tearfully, said, "Mrs. White died last night."

"Yes, I know," I answered; we held hands for just a moment.

"She was such a lovely lady," she added; then she and her husband hurried on. She never thought to introduce me to him.

At the hospice, as a young chaplain-in-training walked down the ward corridor, a nurse who was a member of his support group rushed across in front of him and dashed into the kitchen. As she ran, she mumbled, "Grace just died." Grace had been a young nurse who had come to the hospice with lung cancer; she was a special favorite of all the nurses on the ward.

The chaplain followed the nurse into the kitchen and found her sobbing uncontrollably, sitting with her head buried in her

Staff Support

arms on the table. He felt completely at a loss for words. He put his hand on her shoulder for a minute. Then he left. That afternoon, the nurse came up to him in the coffee room and said, "Thank you for being so kind and sensitive to what I needed most of all in that moment."

"Pump-Primers"

Support groups usually find they need some helps, or "pump-primers," in the early stages of development. Today's openness on the subject of dying has generated a plethora of materials that might be used as discussion-starters for new groups. J. William Worden's *P.D.A.* (Prentice Hall, 1976) and Robert E. Neale's *The Art of Dying* (Harper and Row, 1973) are two books with an abundance of such exercises.

One of the best "primers" is the Life-line. People are asked to draw a line across a sheet of paper. They are then told, "That line is your life." They then place an "x" on the line where they think they are now in their life. Both *chronos* and *kairos* are involved in the decision. The next step is to talk with somebody else about where they have put their "x" and how they went about making their decision. The first time I did this primer exercise, an eighty-two year old lady put her "x" well to the left of center, "Because," she said, "there's so much out there waiting for me."

Another discussion-starter is a series of questions designed to help people clarify their feelings and attitudes about death:

1. About death, I feel
   _ It's best not to think of it
   _ Curious
   _ Scared
   _ It won't happen to me for years
   _ It's something that has to be
2. If I were dying of something incurable, I would rather
   _ Be told what was happening to me
   _ Not to be told about it
3. When I die, I want to be
   _ At home, if possible

– In a hospital
– Conscious as much as possible
– Conscious as little as possible

Another productive exercise is to ask each person to write his or her own obituary. Or, each might be asked:

How often do you think of dying?
What do you dread most about the dying process?
Did you ever lose a pet?
What is your earliest recollection of a funeral?
What are the three most important things in your life?

These and similar pump-priming exercises will facilitate the creation of an open and honest atmosphere among the group's members. This atmosphere will, in turn, enhance the effectiveness of the entire staff support system.

The System Is Right

The staff support system finally pays off in an institutional flexibility that can pick up on an informally presented problem, and open it up as a learning instrument for everyone.

St. Christopher's has a number of people from the Caribbean on its staff. They speak calypso; their speech dances and sparkles. It is captivating, entrancing.

I was mesmerized one day in the coffee room as I listened to Estelle, a lovely nurse from Trinidad, only recently on the hospital staff, tell me about her family. When she concluded, I asked her how she liked working at St. Christopher's. She paused, then surprised me.

"I have been having bad dreams lately," she said.
"What kind of dreams?"
"They're about Alex," came her reply.

Alex was a young man of twenty-three on her ward who had an enormous malignancy on his throat. It looked like a goiter, and was growing wildly. Seven months ago, he had awakened one morning with a sore throat. Now, this! He was having trouble breathing. A tracheotomy was performed, making his respiration a little easier for him.

"In every dream, I see Alex," Estelle continued. "He's strangling. And I wake up in a sweat and cannot get back to sleep."

"How long has this been going on?" I asked.

"For five nights straight," she said, a note of panic in her voice.

"Have you talked with anybody else about this?"

"Oh, no," came her lilting response. "I would not dare tell anybody. I only tell you."

That afternoon I asked the head nurse if she had had any inkling of Estelle's problem. She indicated that she had picked up a hint or two. Now, she said, it seemed time to take action. Several relatively inexperienced nurses worked on Alex's ward; they were probably just as worried about his condition as was Estelle. They were undoubtedly anxious about how Alex would die. Surely, it would seem to those new to hospice techniques that Alex might die an agonizing death, and that they might find themselves standing by, helpless and frustrated.

Within two days, a seminar was arranged for the staff people on Alex's ward. The head nurse was there. The regular chaplain, who had been through this sort of thing numerous times before, was there. Nurses and volunteers and orderlies—some of whom had logged considerable hospice experience—were there. Then there were others, like Estelle, for whom Alex's condition posed the threatening question, "What shall I do if he is strangling?"

The head nurse, the chaplain and others of experience began talking about Alex and about other Alexes who, in the past, had been kept comfortable during their last days and who had died peacefully. When the meeting was over, no one had the slightest doubt that the same peaceful end was awaiting Alex. The doctors would medicate him sufficiently to keep his breathing even.

When Alex died four days later, peacefully, without a trace of struggle, the hospice program of caring was once again vindicated. And the more experienced staff members had provided a helpful kind of support for the newer members. Together, they realized that they all belonged to a system that could not possibly fail, because, at its heart, it was right.

7

Hospice Volunteers

Charles Campbell had been heavily sedated for several weeks when he was finally admitted to St. Christopher's. However, the sedation had lost its effect, had given him no relief from his agonizing pain. With an estimated six weeks to live, he arrived at the hospice on a Tuesday morning. On Wednesday afternoon, while I was making my rounds, I stopped to say hello and get acquainted. "How is St. Christopher's treating you, Mr. Campbell?" I asked.

"Just fine, Chaplain," he replied. "I can't believe it, but I've no pain today; first time in six months that I've not had pain. The food is good here. They don't bother you when you want to be left alone. They answer your questions. If they don't know the answers, they find somebody who does. They sit down and listen. The doctor, the nurses, the orderlies, they're all wonderful. And those nice 'Orange People' are a very special lot."

"Those nice 'Orange People'" are the hospice volunteers. St. Christopher's Hospice has one-hundred-fifty, many of them orange-clad women who work on the wards with the professional staff. In America, where most of the hospice programs to date are primarily home-centered, both staff and volunteers make house calls, but they do not wear orange uniforms.

A core of carefully selected and thoroughly trained volunteers is basic to effective hospice care of the terminally ill and their families. An important hospice goal is to give families an opportunity to establish and maintain a personal relationship with someone on the hospice team. The volunteer provides this opportunity by devoting larger amounts of time to a family than the professional staff can give.

A Rare Breed

Hospice volunteers are truly exceptional human beings. Their response, loyalty, sincerity and commitment are so unusual that one expert with years of experience in working with volunteers said, "You can throw away the book when it comes to hospice volunteers. You don't have to keep them busy to hold their interest. They have an amazing willingness to be inconvenienced. Their appetite for learning is insatiable. The satisfaction derived from their service seems to come easily and often to them. And their commitment runs deep." The last sentence is the clincher. The Connecticut Hospice, for example, recruited and trained forty-six volunteers in one year. Of that number, ten dropped out, but all left for reasons other than lack of interest or commitment.

People volunteer their services in our society for a variety of reasons: they may want to be helpful and useful; they may require the satisfaction of the "thank you" that comes from personal service; they may seek some type of status; they may use their service as an escape; they may hope to land a paying job with the organization; they may want to learn; they may want to put their religious faith into more concrete action. Perhaps the most effective and reliable volunteers are those whose misfortune has motivated them to aid other people with similar afflictions. Organizations of parents who have leukemic children and relatives of those stricken with multiple sclerosis are good examples of motivation to serve others.

Hospice volunteers may also be motivated by the priceless opportunity to learn about the dying process; to learn about courage and dignity and all those other qualities which sound ridiculous and hackneyed until you see them in action; to learn about the importance of saying "I love you" and "Goodbye"; to learn about the all-rightness of death. There is something magnetically heroic about the struggle to find meaning and beauty in the fleeting last days of one's life. To be responsible, in some way, for enabling that beauty and meaning to flourish is to share in the heroism of the experience. To hold a hand in the last moments is to experience the holiest of mysteries. It is to stand at the point where two worlds touch.

At a meeting of widows in a local church, a woman spoke lovingly of her husband's lengthy battle with cancer. She told of his wasting away, of his fighting spirit that gave up only a few days before his death, of her sleepless nights and his restless days during the interminable illness, and of the occasional moments of precious tenderness they shared before he mercifully died. At that point, another woman burst out, "Oh, you were so fortunate! My husband died of a heart attack while I was out of town. We never got to say goodbye!" There *is* something very basic to be experienced in the period of terminal illness. And hospice people are enriched from being involved, however slight their involvement may actually be.

Another motivation for the hospice volunteer may be the opportunity to creatively finish their own task of grieving. Bereavement counsellors tell us that guilt feelings are normal in the mourning process, that unfinished business will be found in the wake of every severed relationship. Consequently, helping another patient in another family may very well contribute to a healthy resolution of one's own unfinished business.

An American woman who was living in London temporarily and had volunteered her services to St. Christopher's for one day a week is a case in point. Her own mother, a humorless and demanding woman, had died of cancer five years earlier after a bitter struggle with agonizing pain, in the austere and unattractive surroundings of a modest nursing home. Once a week the woman would don the familiar orange uniform of the St. Christopher's volunteer and assist the nurses and orderlies on the ward. She sat and listened to patients who just wanted to talk. She read to those who wanted to be read to. In her second month of service, she realized that she was spending more time with one particular woman patient than with all the others combined. When she mentioned this friendship to one of the staff, the nurse replied, "It's wonderful. You're the only person who can relate to her. Everyone else finds her abrasive and unduly demanding, but you seem to understand and accept her." The volunteer then realized that her experience at St. Christopher's was a replay of her mother's ordeal. This time, however, she was far more capable of helping.

One afternoon the volunteer told the patient about her own mother, about how similar her mother and the patient were, about her mother's last days, about how glad she, the volunteer, was to be more helpful now in a hospice setting. The patient's world grew smaller with each day. Her children and grandchildren withdrew. But the dying woman was satisfied to have her new "daughter" near until the end.

People also become hospice volunteers because many of them find in hospice service a means of memorializing a loved one. St. Christopher's derives—and other hospices hope to derive—a substantial income each year from people who are grateful for what the hospice did for their loved one and for themselves. A good many volunteers donate hours of their service for the same reasons.

Many other volunteers offer their time and money because hospice care was not available when someone close to them suffered the agonies of chronic pain during their last days. Now that a new and much-needed way of caring has arrived on the scene—one that assures physical comfort without diminution of lucidity, and which provides technical, medical, social, emotional and spiritual support for the patient and for the family—there are those who offer to help others as a kind of living memorial. And where no hospice is yet in operation, the dreamers and planners receive countless letters and calls offering assistance.

An additional motivation for volunteering service in a hospice program is the simple need to contribute to a system of caring that one may later use oneself. Cancer is a fearsome enemy in our society. Anyone who has had even a casual contact with it knows something not only of physical ordeal but also of emotional exhaustion. The spector of unrelieved pain is truly frightening; threatening is the notion that one may be alone in one's last days, shunned by otherwise caring people who cannot face witnessing a slow and painful death. Consequently, the arrival of a caring system that takes pain and aloneness seriously is a cause of personal relief, if not rejoicing. As one hospice advocate put it: "I have not yet met persons in the hospice movement who did not admit to wanting to contribute to a system which might some day conceivably support them. The motivation is deep. It is personal. And it is legitimate."

The Arm-Proppers

Behind the scenes in any local hospice program is a vast number of people who dedicate their time and money, their skill and energy without any financial compensation. Volunteers far outnumber paid workers, and most of them never come in contact with patients and their families. But without their support, there would be no hospice. Theirs is a classic role, reminiscent of an honored Jewish legend.

The armies of Amalek had challenged Israel at Rephidim. Moses sent Israel into battle with the assurance that God was with them. As they fought, Moses was visible on the hilltop, holding his hands high. So long as he held them up, Israel prevailed. But Moses's arms became weary; when he lowered his hands, the armies of Amalek prevailed. So Moses's aides, Aaron and Hur, propped up Moses's arms during the long battle. Their support enabled Israel to win the day.

Hospice volunteers are the Aarons and the Hurs who support the direct-caregivers. First, there are the interested citizens in the community who, aware of a critical need, see in hospice a way to meet that need. These people band together to establish a local hospice program. They form work and study committees. They draw up bylaws. They incorporate. They negotiate a tax-free status for their charitable organization. They choose boards of directors and charge them with the task of providing hospice services. And what an arduous task it turns out to be! Some hospice programs have taken three to five years to deliver their initial services because the planners want to get the program right. And getting it right means walking—sometimes very slowly—the long and tedious planning route: becoming thoroughly acquainted with hospice theory of care for the terminally ill, becoming acquainted and comfortable with one another, educating the community, spending countless hours enlisting the support of other key persons and agencies, assessing the needs of the community, designing a unique hospice program to meet those community needs, exploring ways to have the cost of hospice services reimbursed, establishing ties with other hospice programs, raising money, and confronting a seemingly endless succession of obstacles. All of these things must be done, and done correctly, while simultaneously coping with a growing frustration over being unable to respond to the calls from families hospice could help—if only a program were in operation.

As planning nears fruition, other volunteers begin their services: newsletter writers and mailers, publicity and information disseminators, fund raisers, hospice librarians, to name just a few. Others offer more specialized gifts. The father of a young woman who died at St. Christopher's still devotes one weekend each month working in the hospice gardens. Another man, whose wife died there, volunteered to keep the hospice ambulance sparkling inside and out. While in a local American hospice, a tropical fish fancier keeps the hospice's aquarium tanks clean and balanced.

Still others volunteer services that will indirectly touch the patients and their families. They serve as house-cleaners, errand-runners and car-drivers, hairdressers, escorts for nurses making house calls in unsafe areas, providers of temporary housing for out-of-town family members, and the like. It is not unusual for the Director of Hospice Volunteers to be a volunteer in that position.

Few volunteers in any given hospice program become intimately involved with patients and their families. But those who do are particularly noteworthy because they lend support to the professional staff as well as to the families. The volunteer will establish close ties with the family by spending more time with them than professional staff possibly can.

Motivated to Care

Hospice volunteers are in the program because they want to be there. No one is coerced into hospice work. Because Cicely Saunders understands that even voluntary participation in a hospice program can be an emotionally exhausting experience, one of her famous guidelines runs, "Don't get into hospice work if you can possibly avoid it." The spirit of that advice permeates the movement, but thousands seem unable to "avoid" becoming involved.

At the same time, not everyone who feels motivated to serve is accepted in a hospice program. A careful screening process is used to select the caregivers who will be accepted into the program from the large number of applicants who sincerely offer their services to the hospice. The screening begins with a lengthy, informal interview, the purpose of which is twofold: first, to help the Director of Volunteers become acquainted with the volunteer and with his or her reasons for applying, and to begin thinking about the ideal position for the volunteer in the program; and second, to help the applicant begin to understand the hospice program and what is expected of a care giving volunteer.

The applicant is asked to touch upon a broad variety of personal issues in the interview. Since most hospice groups discourage people who have recently suffered a significant personal loss from working in the hospice program as direct caregivers, the Director will want to know if a personal loss is the motivation for the person's volunteering his or her services at that time. If it is not, the Director will want to know why the person is volunteering now. The Director will ask questions about the potential volunteer's availability, time commitment, the distance the volunteer will be willing to travel to visit a patient. Volunteers will also respond to questions concerning health, hobbies and interests. They will discuss their family life, their feelings about themselves, and their feelings about seeing bloody sights or smelling foul odors. The Director will have to know the volunteers' attitudes about the dying process, and, perhaps most importantly, their attitude about their own death.

An ongoing screening process is set into motion during the interview. As the volunteer and the Director become acquainted, they learn to trust each other with ideas, evaluations, and opinions. The volunteers find that the hospice program cares about them in a very personal way. They find that they may feel free to opt out of direct care giving at any time, either temporarily or permanently. If this should happen, some hospices go so far as to help a misplaced volunteer find another more suitable position with another agency in the community. The bottom line for the volunteers is that they are part of a caring and supportive system.

Informed about the Program

Every hospice direct-care volunteer understands hospice philosophy, has an overview of the local hospice program, and is conversant with the community resources a patient's family may need.

Volunteers should have the same confidence in the pain-control regimen as the Meidical Director and the Director of Nursing have.

Volunteers should view the entire family as the primary unit of caring.

Volunteers should be aware of the need to be both gentle and realistic in the face of impending death.

Volunteers must see themselves as part of an interdisciplinary team that knows how to support one another.

Volunteers will understand something of the medical, emotional, social, and spiritual needs of dying persons which the hospice movement attempts to meet.

The Problem in the Beginning

When hospice volunteer trainees are asked how they view the way in which our society usually deals with a terminal illness, their answers pour forth out of personal experience:

—Everybody is "cool." Nobody makes a fuss. Death just happens and nobody is bothered much.
—Very few people are involved, the fewer the better; health care institutions discourage visiting and prohibit children from the scene.
—There are no rituals, no formal goodbyes.
—The doctor's involvement decreases; the chaplain's visits increase.
—The focus is on the patient's physical needs; little

effort is made to accommodate the needs of the family who are discouraged from visiting because "there is nothing you can do."
—After the patient's death, the family is expected to be grateful for the "best medical care in the world," and they are largely ignored a few days after the funeral.
—The family goes home; business as usual.

Volunteers will learn about the hospice idea of caring that attempts to meet those patient and family needs which our society and our medical system largely ignores. They will learn that each patient has unique needs, that these needs are based upon a unique lifestyle and way of coping with crises, and that the uniqueness of the person must be of paramount concern to the caregiver. Volunteers will learn that control of the patient's pain is an utmost priority, that if they don't care about the patient's pain, they don't care about the patient. Volunteers will learn that every effort must be made to keep the patient comfortable.

Other basic principles of the hospice theory of care for the terminally ill will be impressed upon the volunteers during their training program:

> —The patient's wishes regarding prolongation of life when no recovery is possible must be honored.
> —The patient and the family have the right to discuss openly and together the patient's condition if they wish to.
> —The patient and family must be in control of the surroundings as much as possible; they, and not the institution or the caregivers, should determine who visits the patient and when.
> —The family has the right to determine how they will take leave of the one who is dying and how they will mark the event when death occurs.
> —The family's need for support continues after the patient has died.

Meeting the Needs

The primary question facing the recruited volunteer is "How does the local hospice try to meet these needs?" The answer is supplied in several ways. For one thing, all hospices include in their training program an extensive orientation in hospice philosophy and the way the local hospice works. Then, too, many hospice programs provide a period of apprenticeship during which the volunteer may accompany a staff person in home visitation. Such visits are followed by recap sessions in which such subjects as (1) What happened during the visit? (2) What patient and family needs were expressed? (3) Did we help them? (4) Where did we fail? (5) How did you feel during the visit? are discussed at length. Thus, volunteers learn by experience and by reflection.

Volunteers also learn by being included in meetings when professional staff members discuss the families to whom they have been assigned. In addition to learning more about the family's needs, the volunteers gradually put together the pieces of the local hospice operation: Who answers the phone nights and weekends? Who makes house calls? Who plays the consultant's role? How do team members, including the volunteers, relate to each other? These and countless other questions are answered, slowly yet surely, during the training and apprenticeship parts of the program.

Providing salient information to the families as they request it is another aspect of the local program about which volunteers learn. And these requests can sometimes catch one off-balance. For one thing, there are anticipatory needs. A patient, looking ahead, may suddenly announce that he is making funeral plans: he wants to be cremated; he wants a memorial service at the yacht club; he wants his ashes strewn around Pigeon Point Lighthouse, and so on. Then he asks such questions as "Does a person have to be embalmed in order to be cremated?" and "How inexpensively can I be buried?" A well informed volunteer will either have the answers to the questions or know where to find them.

The man's wife, meantime, may also be anticipating some problems. If her husband does not want to have his life unnecessarily prolonged, and if both of them want him to die at home, there are already some existing guidelines for her. But what if she panics in the heat of a crisis? That was Margaret McKenzie's concern.

Margaret's husband "Mac" wanted to die at home, and the hospice team was helping her care for him. One day she said to the hospice volunteer, "I wonder if I'll be able to keep him here if there's a crisis? I know that if I called an ambulance and had him taken to the hospital, they would do their best to keep him alive; that's their job, but it's not what "Mac" and I want. Still, I don't know if I'll be able to handle it." The volunteer listened, repeated again some options open to her in a crisis situation such as calling the volunteer or the hospice Medical Director or the neighbor who was a nurse, and offered a reassuring "Whatever you do, it will be because you love him."

The crisis came for "Mac" and Margaret. They were alone when "Mac" began coughing up blood. Margaret waited for a couple of hours, then called the hospice Medical Director.

"Should I take him to the hospital?" she asked.

"If you wish," the doctor replied. "I can call the ambulance for you."

"What will they do to him there?"

"They will give him a blood transfusion, more than likely."

"Thank you Doctor. You're very helpful. I knew that, but I guess I just needed to hear you say it. We'll manage all right at home."

Margaret went back to her husband, resumed cleaning him up as best she could, then held him close. "Mac" died in her arms. And she recalls, wistfully yet triumphantly, that he gave her a faint smile and a wink just before he died.

The focus of Margaret's story is not so much on her decision as on the support she received from the volunteer who offered appropriate information and reassurance. Many another Margaret has decided to call the ambulance for her "Mac," and has sat close to him in the hospital in those last moments. And many another "Mac" has smiled and winked in just the same way. And many another hospice caregiver has said to those Margarets, "You were magnificent! I'm so proud of you!"

When It's Over

What happens when a patient dies at home? Whom does the spouse call? The rescue squad? The police? The doctor? The funeral director? A neighbor? The minister? This is the type of questioning a hospice volunteer can anticipate. The answers, in many instances, are locally determined and a hospice volunteer can be an immediate help by being well informed. The answer to "What do I do now?" is usually similar to the following suggested procedure:

> (1) Call the doctor. He or she will come to the house, sign and leave the death certificate. Give the doctor three to four hours to arrive.
> (2) If you cannot locate the doctor, call the police department.
> (3) The body cannot be removed from the house until the Medical Examiner gives the order either to have the body removed by a funeral director or to have an autopsy performed. Again, allow the Medical Examiner an hour or so to arrive.
> (4) Notify a funeral director who will then remove the body and set an appointment with the family to make funeral arrangements. Many funeral directors strongly recommend that the children in the family be included in the decision making process as much as possible.

The time between the patient's death and the doctor's arrival may seem an eternity. If hospice has been involved, the spouse will probably want to inform one of the caregivers of the patient's death. That caregiver is often the volunteer. When called, the hospice person will find a way to come to the house as soon as possible, and will stay with the family as long as the presence of a friend is needed.

Hospice care includes great respect for and tenderness toward the body of the deceased person. A well informed and deeply caring volunteer, offering to help bathe the body or participating in a family prayer at the bedside or simply saying a verbal "Goodbye" can be a blessing to the family in the interminable period between the moment of death and the beginning of official processing.

Hospice volunteers are, therefore, thoroughly informed about hospice philosophy and about how the local hospice program functions. Their introduction is thorough, and their training is vigorous.

Trained to be Helpful

If you were terminally ill, what kind of person would you most want to visit with you? One local hospice group asked that question of themselves as they began designing a training program for volunteers. Their answers provided a broad outline for their design. "I would like a person who . . .

> took time to sit with me
> was a good listener
> helped me keep my pride and self-respect
> maintained confidentiality
> was trustworthy, dependable, patient
> respected and championed my rights as a patient
> helped my family and me to maintain as much control as possible over the situation
> heard me and responded appropriately; laughed with me, cried with me
> accepted me totally, was not upset by my physical appearance or limitations
> was comfortable with herself or himself
> was comfortable with silence and with touching
> was aware of her or his own limitations
> was enthusiastic and enjoyed life
> was realistic about death
> could support us without needing *our* support
> was unbiased, non-judgmental
> would remain a friend to my family after I died
> could help me live until I died."

To meet all these needs all the time is, of course, impossible. But hospice tries, and keeps on trying. Hospice wants its volunteer caregivers not only to be helpful, but to be a credit to the whole hospice movement as well. As the president of one local hospice movement put it, "We screen our volunteers carefully, train them arduously, and support them continuously because, frankly, we never want hospice to be an embarrassment to the community."

Careful screening means about a two-hour application interview, a review of one's involvement as a caregiver during the training period, a lengthy post-training interview, and ongoing participation in the staff support system.

The actual training program of each hospice is unique in its design. It may be anywhere from ten to twenty-five hours long, and the training techniques may vary from group to group. But all hospice trainees learn skills that translate hospice philosophy into personal care giving. Some instructors recommend mottos, or catch phrases, or "handles" that will later suggest to the volunteer some broader concepts of care giving. "Handles" like the following also give the patient and family some ideas about the qualifications of the hospice volunteer.

Listen Loudly

Listening is a skill. Like all skills, it is nurtured through regular practice. Hospice training sessions are liberally sprinkled with opportunities for learning to listen with the heart and mind as well with the ear, to "listen loudly," as one hospice caregiver put it. No single requirement of a hospice caregiver is greater than the ability to listen. The renowned Quaker leader, Douglas Steere, was correct when he equated listening to loving. If you love someone, you will listen to that person. If you do not listen, you do not love.

Many lives have been saved, and many have been changed because someone listened at the right time. That is especially true for a person who is living under the stress of loss, both actual and pending. Sooner or later, all hospice caregivers receive a phone call from the spouse of a patient or from a widow that catches them off-guard. One caregiver offers the following experience:

> My phone at home rang one night at 10:30. It was Mrs. J. whose husband had died four months before. I was tired and out of sorts. My wife and I had patched up an argument and had just gone to bed. My initial feeling about the phone call was one of resentment. I wanted to tell Mrs. J. to take two aspirin and call me in the morning. But I couldn't break into her tearful monologue. She had been coping so beautifully, she said. Now, she was sure she would never be able to live without her husband.

She sobbed as though there would be no tomorrow for her, and she went on for about half an hour. I felt increasingly helpless and frustrated. When she hung up, I wondered what I could or should have said to her.

Next evening, at about 7:30, Mrs. J. called again. She was chipper, amusing, confident. She said merely, "Thanks so much for being there and just listening to me. I'll be all right. I'll make it now, I'm sure of it."

The lesson is taught again and again: listening is the gift of the helpful, not the futility of the helpless. And while listening may be all that is asked of us, it is nonetheless the greatest gift we can give and the noblest tribute we can bestow.

Find Out

Frank Laubach, former missionary, educator, and creator of the "each-one-teach-one" scheme which has upgraded literacy throughout the entire Third World, had a simple motto which described his service goals: "Find out what a person needs and give it to him; find out what he is proud of and praise him for it." That motto succinctly expresses the hospice caregivers task—*find out*.

In order to "find out" what the patient and family need, one must be open and unbiased. The idea is for the volunteer to enter any new helping relationship as a clean slate, inviting patients and families to "write down," in a sense, who they are, what they need, and what they hope for. To "find out" is to determine and to encourage the family's control over their situation. To "find out" is to let them decide who will visit and when and for how long, or how the family members will relate to the patient right up to the very end, whether in the home or in the hospital. The family should be asked their advice rather than be told what they must do next.

The volunteer caregiver will have ample opportunity to give honest praise to the patient and the family. It is not necessary to manufacture it. A patient may talk about his grandchildren, or his professional or athletic or academic achievements. He may mention "the forty years of our happy marriage." The patient needs to be praised for what he is proud of, and for his present courage. He does not need to be reminded of his failures or his shortcomings.

At the same time, his spouse needs a pat on the back for the way she is weathering her storm. She may not be caring for her husband and her family the way the volunteer thinks she should be caring for them in that situation; but she is doing some positive things, and the caregiver will accentuate those positives and will praise her for whatever she has been able to accomplish.

Hands On . . . Hands Off

Volunteers are carefully instructed not to attempt to perform any of the duties of professionals, like the nursing staff, for instance. At the same time, the volunteer is a friend to the family. Being a friend implies affection and appropriate spontaneity. All hospice people try to walk the line between propriety and spontaneity. They will all fluff a pillow or hold a hand when it seems called for, but they do not overstep the boundaries of their defined responsibilities.

Promises, Promises

As one tries to be helpful in the heat of a stressful crisis, one is tempted to make promises that cannot or will not be kept. More than likely the one to whom the promises are made, the victim in the tragedy, will grasp at the straw of the promises and will desperately believe that they will be kept. The later disappointment over not having the promises kept may be monumental.

"You're getting better all the time," says the doctor to the dying man.

"I'll keep in touch," promises the friend who never again calls or visits.

"Call me if there is ever anything I can do . . . anytime, I don't care!" vows the relative who, when called, stumbles and stammers, "Gee, I can't do it today. How about next Tuesday?"

"Oh, John, I promise I'll be there with you when you die!" pledges the dedicated caregiver.

It may be a trifling thing, that unkept promise, and under normal circumstances it would be understood and manageable. But there is nothing "normal" about the circumstances surrounding the dying person and his family. In those most unusual circumstances, the unkept promise sometimes feels like total abandonment. Consequently, in their training program, hospice volunteers are steeped in the importance of "Promising only what you can deliver, and delivering everything you promise." Recipients of hospice care should know, then, that when the volunteer says, "Call me any time you want to talk," the around-the-clock promise to listen is a bona fide offer that will be honored.

The belief that in order to die with dignity a person should have someone at the bedside at the time of death is well intentioned but unrealistic. No one, not even a spouse, can be sure that she or he will be present at that very moment. "I'll be with you" is, therefore, a promise whose keeping lies beyond human management. Besides, there is a touch of superstition in the suggestion that the dying person was deprived of a proper send-off if no one was holding his hand when he died.

At St. Christopher's, most patients die during the night when there is no one sitting at the bedside. No one on the staff feels indadequate or defeated by that fact. "There's nothing wrong with dying alone," commented one chief ward nurse. "People have been doing it for years. Besides," she added, "no one is actually alone in this place. We are all surrounded by love here, patients and staff alike, and we know it whether we're with somebody or alone."

Of all the people involved, the patient best understands the emptiness of the promise "I'll be with you when you die." The husband of a dying woman said that he really didn't want to go out of the house, despite his wife's insistence that he get a change of scenery. "I want to stay close," he said. To which his wife replied, "But how close is close?" She understood, far better than anyone else, that ultimately she was alone.

You're Leaving, I'm Staying

Humility is something a hospice caregiver learns with experience. And awe. They also learn respect for the members of the family who are carrying the burden of a pending loss of life and love.

Hospice volunteers are taught to *try* to understand, but never to claim actually *to* understand. To say to a dying man or to his spouse "I understand" is a ridiculous superficiality which broadens the emotional gap that already exists between the family and the rest of the world, a gap that can never finally be spanned. Better to say nothing than to say "I understand."

One patient described the gap to the hospice caregiver who had visited him faithfully over a period of months when he told her, "Charlotte, I always enjoy your visits. When I'm down, you pick me up. When I'm up, you laugh with me. I appreciate your ideas and your thoughts. You're a stimulating person. You're a good friend. But let's face it. When you walk out of that door, I'm still in this bed."

To honor the unbridgeable gap that exists between the dying person and all others is to be humbled and awed by a great mystery.

Patients Are Not Equal

The entire training focus regarding the dying patient and the family is that each person and each family is unique in all the world. The family's coping mechanisms are singularly their own. It is the task of the volunteer caregiver both to identify and to respect that uniqueness. Respect means never violating the special style of the family facing a crisis. No human being has the right to destroy another's defenses. Every person has the right, finally, to die with either dignity or indignity, as he wishes. Every person has the right to live by denial if he wishes. His style is his own, and hospice volunteers are trained to respect that style.

This point was well made, with both a touch of humor and a volume of realism, by one trainer of volunteers. He told the group about his young son who had been stricken mysteriously and seriously. No one could be at all certain of the prognosis. Someone in the group asked him if he were not preoccupied with his son's condition all the time. "No, not always," replied the trainer. "When I'm at home, of course, he is the center of our lives. But when I go to work, I can actually forget about him. If I couldn't, I think I'd crack wide open." Then he added, "Thank God for denial!" That's the way this man was coping with his personal crisis.

The Marathon

In the parlance of the Olympic Games, hospice would be a sprint if it were involved only with the relatively brief period before the patient's death. But a volunteer's commitment to a family continues well after the patient has died. Bereavement is long and arduous. The hospice commitment, then, is a marathon effort, and volunteer caregivers are trained for the long distance run.

The volunteer's sights need to be set on at least a full year of touching base with the widowed family, especially during the holidays, on birthdays and anniversaries, and other special occasions. The widowed person never knows what effect those occasions will have upon a lonely life until the day or season actually arrives.

Joseph M. died on March 19th. His wife, according to a close friend, was managing quite well in her bereavement. She and her children had some difficulty during their "first Christmas without Dad," but they had bounced back again with resilience and confidence. It was on the following February 13th, the Eve of St. Valentine's Day, that she called a hospice volunteer with whom she had not talked since the holidays, "Just to talk," she said, "because all of a sudden I am wondering if I can make it through Valentine's Day. You see, it was always a special day for Joe and me. We met at a Valentine party; and after we were married, we went out for dinner together each year on Valentine's Day." She paused, the added, "I know it sounds silly, but he always called me his Valentine, and...."

She did get through the crisis, of course, the crisis not only of Valentine's Day but of the calendar year as well, that yearly round of family rituals that would never again be quite the same for her.

Weep Some, Laugh Some

Once it has been established that tears and laughter are valid and legitimate means of communication, even in the sickroom, appropriate emotional responses can be learned by the hospice volunteer. The ancient biblical admonition to "weep with those who weep and rejoice with those who rejoice" applies to the hospice caregiver. There are times when a tear will communicate the personal concern and caring for which the patient may have been starving. Indeed, when a caregiver is compassionate, tears "in the right places" are almost inevitable, for tears are vehicles for communicating an intimate part of one's humanity to another human being.

The same is true of laughter, although humor is rarer than tears in the presence of a person who lies dying. The appropriateness of humor depends almost completely upon the patient and the family. If humor is in the family fabric, volunteers' responsive humor can add immeasurably to the family's emotional resources.

If patients have a sense of humor, they have something very special going for them. If they try to share their humor, they will want it appreciated. One man, for example, greeted a volunteer one day with, "Guess what! I just read about Kubla Khan's Five Stages of Dying!" Happily, the volunteer had also read Kübler-Ross' book and thus caught the twinkle in his eye.

A widow needs someone to laugh with her as she relates what she feels are the silly things that have been happening to her since her husband's death. One woman spoke over morning coffee in her kitchen about a significant change in her behavior: "Warren was so messy," she began. "I could leave the house in immaculate order, be gone for half an hour, and find it cluttered up again when I returned. I could count on it. But a strange thing happened after he died. I would leave a neat house, and when I returned it was still neat! So, do you know what I do now? I leave it a little bit messy when I go out so it seems more like home when I come back. Isn't that wild?"

The humor most difficult to appreciate is the joke of which you are the butt. Being able to laugh at oneself is a rare gift that can sometimes provide comic relief for all.

Reverend Williams was asked by one of his parishioners to visit her mother, Mrs. Ralph Stanford, who lived with her. Six months earlier, Mrs. Stanford had suffered a stroke which had left her partially paralyzed. Speech was practically impossible for her. She could manage a grunted yes or no, but the effort required to speak even a single word was too great for her. She sat in her chair most of the day and watched television. Occasionally, her daughter could coax a twinkle from her mother, but other than that Mrs. Stanford sat as expressionless as a stoic.

According to her daughter, Mrs. Stanford had written on a pad that she wanted to be baptized, which was why Reverend Williams had been asked to come to the house. When the minister arrived, the daughter showed him into her mother's room, introduced them, left the room and closed the door. Mrs. Stanford looked steely-eyed at Reverend Williams as he asked her, "Do you renounce your sin and the evil that is in the world?" Mrs. Stanford grunted and nodded her assent. "Do you wish to be baptized into the Christian faith?" Again, a grunt. At that point, Reverend Williams took the filled glass that was standing next to a bowl on the end table and poured the contents into the bowl. He then proceeded to baptize Mrs. Stanford, offered a prayer of thanksgiving and praise, and concluded with the benediction. Then he left.

Several days later, Reverend Williams met the daughter at a church function and asked if her mother were pleased at having been baptized. With that, the daughter began an uncontrollable chuckle. "I'm glad you asked, Reverend," she laughed. "You see, when I went back into her room after you left, I asked Mom, 'Did Reverend Williams baptize you?' Mom grunted 'yes.' 'Are you pleased about the baptism?' I asked. Then mom squared her shoulders and spoke, 'Yes. But the damned fool used my 7-Up!' "

Happily, Reverend Williams laughed heartily. But not all counsellors and caregivers do. The sensitivity that can appreciate and respond to the humor of the human drama takes time and effort to develop.

The Finished Product

When hospice volunteers enter a home or a hospital room, one may be certain, then, that they are motivated, informed, and well trained. The volunteer will have a broad understanding of the hospice philosophy and of the local hospice's program and goals.

know about community resources available to the family

be informed of the special attitudes and techniques essential to hospice care, with emphasis on control of chronic pain.

be aware of his or her own mortality, and be comfortable with personal feelings about illness, death, and loss.

have a heightened awareness of the plight of the dying and the patient's family.

have learned skills that can help a family cope with their stress.

be aware of the levels of interpersonal communication.

have practiced basic skills in being helpful to the terminally ill patient and family.

have learned how to be supportive of one who is grieving.

8

Some Final Thoughts About Hospices in America

How To Locate The Nearest Hospice Program

Hospice groups and programs are springing up all across the country. What is happening in Massachusetts is illustrative of the rapid spread of the hospice movement practically everywhere in the United States. In 1977, there was only one incorporated hospice organization, Hospice of Massachusetts, in the state; their Board of Directors was designing a program for the Boston area. Three years later, a new Hospice Federation of Massachusetts included over twenty hospice organizations from around the state, only a few of which were offering services but all of which would be in operation shortly.

Every hospice group is in some way unique; each has designed services which best meet the needs of the community they want to serve. Some include inpatient services. Some are home-care programs. Some are both. There are programs which are related to existing health care agencies. Others are free-standing and independent. Still others serve as an umbrella for existing health care agencies, coordinating and upgrading the community's resources for the terminally ill and their families. But though they may differ in their services and programs, they are one in their espousal of the philosophy of hospice care.

Each hospice group limits its program to a manageable geographical area; that usually means a half-hour travel radius. How, then, does one go about finding the nearest hospice program? I would suggest the following order of search:

Look in the Telephone Directory under "Hospice." Most hospices intentionally incorporate with "Hospice" the first word in their name.

Ask a local minister, rabbi, or priest. Churches and temples are almost always involved in the development of local hospice programs from the outset.

Call the Visiting Nurse Association in your community. They are another community group which participates in the planning.

Contact the Social Services Department in your community hospital. At least one person in that office should know about the hospice efforts in the community.

Ask your doctor. Chances are, however, that if none of the above knows about a local hospice program, neither will your doctor.

For further information about the hospice movement in America, write:

> National Hospice Organization
> 1311A Dolley Madison Blvd.
> McLean, Virginia 22101

Be Sure It's Hospice

Those who have been in the hospice movement for awhile are both pleased and alarmed by the proliferation of hospice programs. They are pleased because this much-needed service is being offered so broadly. They are alarmed by the vast number of community institutions and agencies that, while claiming to be hospices, are something less than the genuine article. Like instant coffee, they are produced in a flash, the consistency determined by personal fancy for immediate satisfaction. One such "hospice" is a nice, clean home for the dying. But this "hospice" offers no medically-directed program for the control of chronic pain, no involvement with patients' families; it maintains a cheerful atmosphere that denies the grim realities of the dying process and adds guilt to the dying patient's baggage because he can't seem to "cheer up"; it provides no bereavement follow-through to the family; there is no deliberate concern for the emotional well-being of the staff.

People in the movement hope for something more consistent, more identifiable, more reliable. They want to insure, for everyone who needs its resources, the integrity of the name "Hospice," so that it stands for and delivers the same basic services everywhere. Consequently, nationally, regionally, and locally the hospice movement is pressing for a body of accepted standards and definitions of purpose which will assure quality control and, at the same time, encourage flexibility and creativity to meet unique local needs.

Those who need its resources, then, can be fairly certain of full hospice services if the local program is affiliated with other hospice groups in the community, in the state, in the nation.

When Searching For A Hospice

What should you look for, then, in a hospice program? Here are a few questions you can ask of the local hospice to help you determine whether or not to use their services.

> (a) Is this an independent, autonomous, non-profit program? A genuine hospice program has its own Board of Directors which determines its own goals and policies. It may very well work through other agencies, perhaps occupying a number of beds in an inpatient facility, for example. But the essential criterion is autonomy, the freedom to determine and to implement policy.
>
> (b) Is there a Medical Advisor for the hospice program? Hospice means first, last, and always, good medical care. Consequently, it is essential to have an M.D. on the staff.
>
> (c) Does the hospice program incorporate a regimen for the control of chronic pain? For those suffering from intractable pain, it is important to know there is someone who cares about the pain, who attempts to control it while enabling the patient to remain lucid and who stays close enough to the situation to be able to change the medication when change is needed.
>
> (d) Does the program offer 24-hour contact service? If there is the slightest hedging on this question,

beware. A genuine hospice program always has around-the-clock telephone service built into it. The contact service means that someone will always be available to listen. Hospice is reliably there.

(e) Is the program interdisciplinary? Interdisciplinary means that the entire program is coordinated. In a legitimate hospice program, you get more than assorted opinions from a variety of professionals. You get a whole team working with you and for you; all the team members hear your requests and try to help meet your specific needs, while simultaneously maintaining an overview of the situation.

(f) How does the program help the family after the patient dies? Bereavement concerns are not immediately paramount to a family when they request hospice services. But they will be. So it pays to learn ahead of time whether or not the program ends when the patient has died. Bereavement follow-up is an integral part of any true hospice program.

Confidentiality

Users of hospice services may be certain that the whole team will observe strict confidentiality. That point is so paramount that it needs to be emphasized. All hospice personnel—staff members and volunteers—are charged not to discuss hospice matters outside hospice meetings. In their attempt to gain the most sensitive assessment of the family's needs, team members will, of necessity, discuss those needs together. But absolute secrecy is maintained once outside the walls of the program. This secrecy is obviously meant to protect the family. But it is also meant to protect the person in whom a patient or a family member has confided. As one patient said to a hospice volunteer, "I don't tell many people that I've had enough." He still needed backing for his pride, and support from the select few who shared his secret.

The Cost Of Hospice Services

It is the strong contention of its proponents that hospice

support can appreciably lower the cost of dying in America. A well-organized home-care program, for instance, that coordinates the services of existing agencies such as Visiting Nurse Association and includes a number of trained volunteers will be considerably less expensive than hospital care. Even if home-care becomes too burdensome for the family, a freestanding and independent inpatient facility will still cost a good deal less than a hospital, but probably a bit more than a nursing home because of the specialized care required.

The actual cost of hospice care is still largely speculative in this country. Third-party insurers, including the Federal Government, are still assessing the hospice movement. They are collecting data to determine if hospice does, indeed, meet heretofore unmet needs, and to determine the degree to which hospices actually lower the cost of terminal care. The Federal Government has awarded two-year pilot grants to twenty-six hospice programs. At the same time, in many states various private insurers, like Blue Cross, are conducting their own pilot studies. At the end of these studies, the cost of hospice services will be much clearer. Future participation in paying for hospice expenses by the government and by private insurers will be determined then.

The dream of hospice people that all persons needing and wanting hospice care will be provided those services, regardless of their ability to pay for them, is a long way from realization. In England, the costs are covered for everyone through the National Health Service. In our country, it would appear that even with Federal Medicare and Medicaid for some, and with private insurers picking up the tab for others, a reservoir of private funds for those not covered by any system will still be necessary. Thus, private foundations, many of which are playing a significant role in the initial period of most hospices, will be needed later on as well, so that no one is ever deprived of quality and humane health care in their last days.

At the present time, then, many health insurance policies cover some aspects of hospice care. Those who desire hospice services will find that hospice personnel are helpful in determining just what kind of health coverage applies in their situation.

For Those Who Need It Most

Finally, hospice care is not for everybody. It is actually for a very small percentage of people. It is an extension of our society's health care system to those for whom the decision to end all treatment of their disease has been made and who, feeling abandoned by that system, reach out for the skill and compassion which seemed all but lost. They may indeed be relatively few in number. But for them, for those who need it most, today and in all our tomorrows, *Hospice Means Hope*!

Kenneth Wentzel, born and educated in the Midwest, seems always to have been identified with innovation. His first postgraduate job took him to Germany in 1947 as a relief coordinator under the then new Church World Service.

For the next 25 years, as a parish minister in Indiana, Maryland and Rhode Island, he was active in emerging social concerns. A self-styled "moderate liberal" he was chairman of the Montogomery County Commission of Human Relations in the early 60's, the first government-sponsored civil rights group in Maryland.

At the same time, he was working on committees toward the merger of his own denomination (Evangelical and Reformed) and the Congregational Christian Churches into The United Church of Christ.

In the mid-60's, he was introduced to the human potential movement, and has since distinguished himself as a leader of small groups, particularly as a viable part of parish activity.

In 1974, he was Visiting Chaplain at St. Christopher's Hospice, London, an experience that led him to devote the next three years to the organization of Hospice Care of Rhode Island, Inc.

Ken Wentzel is, in the words of one of his colleagues, "contageously enthusiastic." An articulate speaker (one longtime parishioner says, "I never heard a dull sermon from Ken Wentzel"), he finds time outside his duties as minister of the Pleasant Street Congregational Church in Arlington, Massachusetts, to speak on the hospice movement and to serve as President of Hospice Care, Inc.

By his own lament, there are too many exciting things to do and to see. "My garden has lots of weeds. My tennis game is rusty. And the fish are running!"

L R C

009170296

91702